Patient Safety

Editor

FEIBI ZHENG

SURGICAL CLINICS OF NORTH AMERICA

www.surgical.theclinics.com

Consulting Editor
RONALD F. MARTIN

February 2021 • Volume 101 • Number 1

ELSEVIER

1600 John F. Kennedy Boulevard • Suite 1800 • Philadelphia, Pennsylvania, 19103-2899

http://www.surgical.theclinics.com

SURGICAL CLINICS OF NORTH AMERICA Volume 101, Number 1
February 2021 ISSN 0039–6109, ISBN-13: 978-0-323-77628-8

Editor: John Vassallo, j.vassallo@elsevier.com
Developmental Editor: Nicole Congleton

Surgical Clinics of North America (ISSN 0039–6109) is published bimonthly by Elsevier Inc., 360 Park Avenue South, New York, NY 10010-1710. Months of publication are February, April, June, August, October, and December. Business and Editorial Offices: 1600 John F. Kennedy Blvd., Suite 1800, Philadelphia, PA 19103-2899. Periodicals postage paid at New York, NY and additional mailing offices. Subscription prices are $443.00 per year for US individuals, $1198.00 per year for US institutions, $100.00 per year for US & Canadian students and residents, $547.00 per year for Canadian individuals, $1270.00 per year for Canadian institutions, $536.00 for international individuals, $1270.00 per year for international institutions and $250.00 per year for foreign students/residents. To receive student/resident rate, orders must be accompanied by name of affiliated institution, date of term, and the *signature* of program/residency coordinator on institution letterhead. Orders will be billed at individual rate until proof of status is received. Foreign air speed delivery is included in all *Clinics* subscription prices. All prices are subject to change without notice. POSTMASTER: Send address changes to *Surgical Clinics*, Elsevier Health Sciences Division, Subscription Customer Service, 3251 Riverport Lane, Maryland Heights, MO 63043. **Customer Service (orders, claims, online, change of address): Telephone: 1-800-654-2452 (U.S. and Canada); 314-447-8871 (outside U.S. and Canada). Fax: 314-447-8029. E-mail: journalscustomerservice-usa@elsevier.com (for print support); journalsonlinesupport-usa@elsevier.com (for online support).**

Reprints. For copies of 100 or more, of articles in this publication, please contact the Commercial Reprints Department, Elsevier Inc., 360 Park Avenue South, New York, New York 10010-1710. Tel. 212-633-3874, Fax: 212-633-3820, E-mail: reprints@elsevier.com.

The Surgical Clinics of North America is also published in Spanish by McGraw-Hill Interamericana Editores S.A., P.O. Box 5-237 06500 Mexico D.F. Mexico; and in Portuguese by Interlivros Edicoes Ltda., Rua Comandante Coelho 1085, CEP 21250, Rio de Janeiro, Brazil; and in Greek by Paschalidis Medical Publications, Athens Greece.

The Surgical Clinics of North America is covered in *MEDLINE/PubMed (Index Medicus), EMBASE/Excerpta Medica, Current Contents/Clinical Medicine, Current Contents/Life Sciences, Science Citation Index*, and *ISI/BIOMED*.

Printed in the United States of America.

Contributors

CONSULTING EDITOR

RONALD F. MARTIN, MD, FACS
Colonel (Retired), United States Army Reserve, Woolwich, Maine

EDITOR

FEIBI ZHENG, MD, MBA, FACS
Assistant Professor of Surgery, Weill Cornell Medical College, Adjunct Assistant Professor of Surgery, Texas A&M, Assistant Member, Houston Methodist Research Institute, Assistant Director of Surgical Quality and Population Health, Department of Surgery, Houston Methodist Hospital, Houston, Texas

AUTHORS

EDWIN ACEVEDO, Jr, MD, MHA
Temple University Lewis Katz School of Medicine, Philadelphia, Pennsylvania, USA

SWARA BAJPAI, MD
Research Resident, Department of Surgery, The University of Alabama at Birmingham, Alabama

BRIAN C. BRAJCICH, MD, MS
Division of Research and Optimal Patient Care, American College of Surgeons, Department of Surgery, Surgical Outcomes and Quality Improvement Center (SOQIC), Northwestern Medicine, Chicago, Illinois

TARA N. COHEN, PhD
Director, Surgical Safety and Human Factors Research, Research Scientist, Assistant Professor, Department of Surgery, Cedars-Sinai Medical Center, Los Angeles, California

FERNANDO RAMIREZ DEL VAL, MD, MPH
Department of Surgery, Houston Methodist Hospital, Houston, Texas

CHELSEA P. FISCHER, MD, MS
American College of Surgeons, Division of Research and Optimal Patient Care, Chicago; Loyola University Medical Center, Maywood, Illinois

BRUCE L. GEWERTZ, MD
Surgeon-in-Chief, H & S Nichols Distinguished Chair in Surgery, Chair, Department of Surgery, Cedars-Sinai Medical Center, Los Angeles, California

AMIR A. GHAFERI, MD, MS
Associate Professor, Department of Surgery, University of Michigan, Ann Arbor, Michigan

ALEX B. HAYNES, MD, MPH
Associate Chair for Discovery and Innovation, Ariadne Labs, Brigham and Women's Hospital, Harvard. T.H. School of Public Health, Boston, Massachusetts; Department of Surgery and Perioperative Care, Dell Medical School, The University of Texas at Austin, Austin, Texas

VANESSA P. HO, MD, MPH
Associate Professor of Surgery and Population and Quantitative Health Sciences, Department of Surgery, MetroHealth Medical Center, Case Western Reserve University School of Medicine, Department of Population and Quantitative Health Sciences, Case Western Reserve University School of Medicine, Cleveland, Ohio

ANGELA INGRAHAM, MD, MS, FACS
Assistant Professor, Department of Surgery, University of Wisconsin-Madison, Madison, Wisconsin

LILLIAN S. KAO, MD, MS
Professor, Jack H. Mayfield, MD, Chair in Surgery, Chief, Division of Acute Care Surgery, Department of Surgery, McGovern Medical School at the University of Texas Health Science Center at Houston, Houston, Texas

AKEMI L. KAWAGUCHI, MD, MS
Associate Professor, Department of Pediatric Surgery, McGovern Medical School at the University of Texas Health Science Center at Houston, Houston, Texas

RACHEL R. KELZ, MD, MSCE, MBA
Vice Chair of Clinical Research, William Maul Measey Professor in Surgery, Department of Surgery, Division of Endocrine and Oncologic Surgery, Center for Surgery and Health Economics, Hospital of the University of Pennsylvania, University of Pennsylvania Perelman School of Medicine, Philadelphia, Pennsylvania

CLIFFORD Y. KO, MD, MS, MSHS, FACS, FSCRS
American College of Surgeons, Division of Research and Optimal Patient Care, Chicago; UCLA Medical Center, Los Angeles, California

LINDSAY E. KUO, MD, MBA
Assistant Professor of Surgery, Temple University Lewis Katz School of Medicine, Philadelphia, Pennsylvania

PRERNA LADHA, MD
Assistant Professor of Surgery, Department of Surgery, MetroHealth Medical Center, Case Western Reserve University School of Medicine, Cleveland, Ohio

ELIZABETH LANCASTER, MD
Resident, Department of Surgery, University of California, San Francisco, California

ALAINA M. LASINSKI, MD
Assistant Professor of Surgery, Department of Surgery, MetroHealth Medical Center, Case Western Reserve University School of Medicine, Cleveland, Ohio

BRENESSA LINDEMAN, MD, MEHP, FACS
Assistant Professor of Surgery and Medical Education, Associate DIO for the Clinical Learning Environment, Department of Surgery, The University of Alabama at Birmingham, Birmingham, Alabama

NIKHIL PANDA, MD, MPH
Resident and Clinical Fellow in Surgery, Department of Surgery, Massachusetts General Hospital, Ariadne Labs, Brigham and Women's Hospital, Harvard. T.H. School of Public Health, Boston, Massachusetts

KEVIN Y. PEI, MD, MHSEd, FACS
Department of Surgery, Houston Methodist Hospital, Houston, Texas

JERICA L. PODRAT, MD
Department of Surgery, Houston Methodist Hospital, Houston, Texas

SHAWN PURNELL, MD, MS
Department of Surgery, Houston Methodist Hospital, Houston, Texas

CAROLINE E. REINKE, MD, MSHP, FACS
Associate Professor, Department of Surgery, Carolinas Medical Center, Atrium Health, Charlotte, North Carolina

CLAIRE B. ROSEN, MD
Resident Physician in General Surgery, Department of Surgery, Division of Surgical Education, Center for Surgery and Health Economics, Hospital of the University of Pennsylvania, Philadelphia, Pennsylvania

DANIEL SHOUHED, MD
Assistant Professor, Department of Surgery, Cedars-Sinai Medical Center, Los Angeles, California

EMILY E. WELLS, MPH
Research Coordinator, Department of Surgery, University of Michigan, Ann Arbor, Michigan

ELIZABETH WICK, MD
Professor, Department of Surgery, University of California, San Francisco, California

FEIBI ZHENG, MD, MBA, FACS
Assistant Professor of Surgery, Weill Cornell Medical College, Adjunct Assistant Professor of Surgery, Texas A&M, Assistant Member, Houston Methodist Research Institute, Assistant Director of Surgical Quality and Population Health, Department of Surgery, Houston Methodist Hospital, Houston, Texas

Contents

Foreword: Patient Safety: Examining Every Aspect of Every System to Improve Outcomes   xiii

Ronald F. Martin

Preface: Captain of the Ship   xvii

Feibi Zheng

A Human Factors Approach to Surgical Patient Safety   1

Tara N. Cohen, Bruce L. Gewertz, and Daniel Shouhed

> This article explores the role of human factors engineering in patient safety in surgery. The authors discuss the history and evolution of human factors and the role of human factors in patient safety and provide a description of human factors methods used to study and improve patient safety.

Teamwork and Surgical Team–Based Training   15

Akemi L. Kawaguchi and Lillian S. Kao

> Effective teamwork, both in and out of the operating room, is an essential component of safe and efficient surgical performance. There are multiple available assessment tools for evaluating teamwork and important contributors to teamwork such as safety culture and nontechnical skills. Multiple types of interventions exist to improve and train providers on teamwork, and many have been demonstrated to improve not only teamwork but also patient outcomes. Teamwork strategies can be adapted to different contexts, based on provider needs and resources.

Processes to Create a Culture of Surgical Patient Safety   29

Claire B. Rosen and Rachel R. Kelz

> This article discusses the processes, interventions, and methods by which health care systems can change the culture of their workplace to promote safety. The importance of this culture shift is discussed, as well as an organizational approach, highlighting the importance of investment of time and resources to the cause. Efforts must include an educational focus on patient safety where a culture of patient safety is emphasized. This attitude along with several specific key interventions, including, measurement, teamwork, briefings, checklists, and developmental infrastructure, are discussed.

Effective Implementation and Utilization of Checklists in Surgical Patient Safety   37

Nikhil Panda and Alex B. Haynes

> The success of patient safety and quality improvement interventions depends, in part, on the effectiveness of implementation. Surgical safety checklists have been introduced into thousands of operating rooms across

6 continents since the debut of the original World Health Organization 19-item checklist in 2008. However, the effect of checklists on patient outcomes has varied. Here, we review 5 examples of large-scale efforts (eg, population level or across health systems) where surgical checklists were introduced into the operating room and the associated effects on patient outcomes. Each experience provides an opportunity to reflect on best practices that inform strategies for effective implementation.

Standardized Care Pathways as a Means to Improve Patient Safety   49

Elizabeth Lancaster and Elizabeth Wick

The literature overwhelmingly supports standardized, evidence-based care to improve patient safety in the surgical setting, including checklists and enhanced recovery programs. Although local culture, patient complexity, and hospital setting can represent barriers to implanting standardized practices, they can be overcome with thoughtful strategies.

Optimizing Safety for Surgical Patients Undergoing Interhospital Transfer   57

Angela Ingraham and Caroline E. Reinke

Interhospital transfers play a key role in ensuring that patients receive necessary care. However, patients who are transferred between hospitals are a vulnerable population, and outcomes of transferred patients are suboptimal. Despite the critical nature of interhospital transfers, only limited effort has been dedicated to standardization and improvement of the transfer process. Studying and adapting quality improvement efforts directed at other transitions of care, particularly those that cross between different facilities and care teams "such as the transition from hospital to home or extended care facilities" may improve the care of surgical patients transferred between acute care institutions.

Improving Postoperative Rescue Through a Multifaceted Approach   71

Amir A. Ghaferi and Emily E. Wells

This article provides a better understanding of how interactions and relationships within hospital microsystems affect rescue. Through structured engagement of clinical champions, these rescue improvement tools may decrease rates of secondary and tertiary complications and enhance staff culture, confidence, and competence. The proposed 3-prong approach sheds light on how health care organizations can better sense, cope with, and respond to the unexpected and changing demands presented by clinically deteriorating postsurgical patients. These interventions lay the groundwork for the further development, testing, and implementation of larger scale rescue-focused initiatives, which could have a direct, population-level impact on mortality.

Provision of Defect-Free Care: Implementation Science in Surgical Patient Safety   81

Alaina M. Lasinski, Prerna Ladha, and Vanessa P. Ho

Implementation science is the study of the translation of evidence-based practices to real-world clinical environments. Implementation is measured with specific outcomes including acceptability, adoption, appropriateness, feasibility, fidelity, penetration, sustainability, and implementation cost. There are defined frameworks and models that outline implementation strategies and assist researchers in identifying barriers and facilitators to achieve implementation and conduct implementation research using methods such as qualitative analysis, parallel group, pre-/postintervention, interrupted time series, and cluster or stepped-wedge randomized trials. Deimplementation is the study of how to remove ineffective or unnecessary practices from the clinical setting and is an equally important component of implementation science.

Evolution of Risk Calculators and the Dawn of Artificial Intelligence in Predicting Patient Complications   97

Jerica L. Podrat, Fernando Ramirez Del Val, and Kevin Y. Pei

Risk calculators are an underused tool for surgeons and trainees when determining and communicating surgical risk. We summarize some of the more common risk calculators and discuss their evolution and limitations. We also describe artificial intelligence models, which have the potential to help clinicians better understand and use risk assessment.

Safety of Surgical Telehealth in the Outpatient and Inpatient Setting   109

Shawn Purnell and Feibi Zheng

New telehealth platforms and interventions have proliferated over the past decade and will be further spurred by the COVID-19 pandemic. Emerging literature examines the efficacy and safety of these interventions. Early pilot studies and trials demonstrate equivalent outcomes of telehealth interventions that seek to replace routine postoperative care in low-risk patients who have undergone low-risk surgeries. Studies are underway to evaluate interventions in higher-risk populations undergoing more complex procedures. Tele-ICU platforms demonstrate promise to provide specialized, high-acuity care to underserved areas and may also be used to augment compliance with evidence-based protocols.

Administrative and Registry Databases for Patient Safety Tracking and Quality Improvement   121

Brian C. Brajcich, Chelsea P. Fischer, and Clifford Y. Ko

Acquisition of data on clinical performance is essential to improve outcomes in surgery. Large, national datasets allow hospitals to monitor events involving patient safety, complications, and benchmark against peer hospitals and facilitate quality improvement (QI) development. Although clinical datasets are often preferable, administrative data also have potential for actionable QI. Hospitals should use whatever data resources may be available and be creative in combining data sources for the most clinically meaningful metrics. Although collection of data is essential in understanding the problems an individual hospital is facing, rigorous QI infrastructure is necessary to translate data to action and achieve sustained change.

The Economics of Patient Surgical Safety   135

Edwin Acevedo Jr and Lindsay E. Kuo

> Adverse surgical events are a major cause of morbidity, mortality, and disability worldwide. Serious reportable events, such as wrong site surgery, retained foreign bodies, and surgical fires, are preventable adverse events that have significant consequences. These "never events" are costly to the patient, health care systems, and society and have led to many efforts to reduce their occurrence. However, these costly events still occur, and more research is needed to obtain a better understanding of their causes and how to prevent them.

The Trainee's Role in Patient Safety: Training Residents and Medical Students in Surgical Patient Safety   149

Swara Bajpai and Brenessa Lindeman

> The focus on patient safety offers a new framework not only for delivering health care but also for training physicians. Medical school and surgical graduate medical education must transition to a more holistic approach by teaching technical and nontechnical skills. Formalized safety curricula can be developed by adopting recommended guidelines and content from national and international organizations, existing validated practices of training programs, frequent simulation exercises, and objective evaluation tools.

SURGICAL CLINICS
OF NORTH AMERICA

FORTHCOMING ISSUES

April 2021
Emerging Bariatric Surgical Procedures
Shanu N. Kothari, *Editor*

June 2021
Esophageal Surgery
John A. Federico and Thomas Fabian,
Editors

August 2021
Education and the General Surgeon
Paul J. Schenarts, *Editor*

RECENT ISSUES

December 2020
Endoscopic Surgery
John H. Rodriguez and Jeffrey L. Ponsky,
Editors

October 2020
Rural Surgery
Tyler G. Hughes, *Editor*

August 2020
Wound Management
Michael D. Caldwell and Michael J. Harl,
Editors

SERIES OF RELATED INTEREST

Advances in Surgery
https://www.advancessurgery.com/
Surgical Oncology Clinics
https://www.surgonc.theclinics.com/
Thoracic Surgery Clinics
http://www.thoracic.theclinics.com/

THE CLINICS ARE AVAILABLE ONLINE!
Access your subscription at:
www.theclinics.com

Foreword

Patient Safety: Examining Every Aspect of Every System to Improve Outcomes

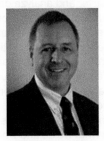

Ronald F. Martin, MD, FACS
Consulting Editor

This issue, Volume 101, Issue 1, marks the beginning of the second century of *Surgical Clinics*. I would be hard-pressed to think of a better topic to begin this new century of sharing information than with Patient Safety. After all, everything we do, everything we learn, everything we teach, and everything we should aspire to, should be for the benefit of the patient. This is why our profession exists.

Safety has become a *loaded* word in recent years. Its meaning has become somewhat obscured and, in some cases, even coopted. One now not only has to consider whether an action, process, or environment is safe but also consider whether it feels safe—and to whom does it feel safe or not. The sociologic discussion of differences of opinion on what constitutes safety and who will be the arbiter of that meaning is beyond capacity and the desire of this foreword. What is necessary for us to examine in our series is what efforts and understandings can we use to make the paths that surgical patients take safer for them to travel. I would like to say that this is a completely objective goal but, there will inherently be some subjectivity, as safety in our context always involves humans, and some of those humans will have differing goals and opinions.

Our concept of safety in the world of surgery has evolved tremendously over the past century. It has not, however, evolved in a vacuum. Nearly every aspect of our lives has evolved its own safety issues as well. Commercial and private transportation, food and water, building codes, clothing, toys, pretty much everything we consume or come in contact with, have some element of scrutiny for safety. Even going to war—arguably one of the least safe things one might contemplate—is replete with safety briefings and equipment (at least in the US Armed Forces).

Surg Clin N Am 101 (2021) xiii–xv
https://doi.org/10.1016/j.suc.2020.09.014
0039-6109/21/© 2020 Published by Elsevier Inc.

surgical.theclinics.com

Safety on some level is a concept, but on another level is a study. The study of what we do and how we apply the knowledge learned from that study in a systematic fashion should allow us all to function in a safer manner. Historically, the concept of surgical practice was that one learned from his/her own mistakes and over time became safer. Beyond that we have Morbidity and Mortality conferences and other meetings that allow us to review our local results and, it is hoped, make improvements, in essence, learn from our own mistakes as well as those of others. A significant category of literature exists on the benefits and drawbacks of learning safety in surgery in this manner.

Improvements in communication and the ability to rapidly transfer and analyze data have allowed us to not only expand our discussions of safety and failure analysis beyond our own walls but also to share concept and techniques with other disciplines. We have been able to share with our colleagues in the flight safety and safety at sea communities to learn very valuable processes. We have been able to share analytical skills and methods with our colleagues in the actuarial and statistical fields. Our colleagues from project management and logistics backgrounds have been able to help us see process issues that have been hindering our best efforts. The list goes on and on.

While the amount that we surgeons can learn from other nonmedical disciplines is nearly limitless, there will always be a major distinction between what we do and what, say, the airline industry must do: in the field of medicine, the end goal is not always agreed upon. If we want to safely fly an aircraft from Logan International Airport in Boston to SeaTac Airport in Washington, we can most assuredly agree on whether the plane took off, traveled, and arrived safely. We may have differing opinions on the comfort of the flight. We may even have room to argue about the safety of the conduct of the crew during the flight in some rare cases, but we almost always could agree on what it meant to have a safely completed flight in terms of moving the aircraft—an aircraft leaves under safe conditions, operates in a safe manner, lands safely at designated destination, and is usable to perform additional flights. When it comes to medicine, we may not be able to agree on the goals of therapy or what constitutes safe performance by the crew, or for that matter when the "flight" is complete. Individual patients and their families ultimately retain the power to make or execute many of the decisions in medicine. In aviation, the passengers don't have that authority. In addition, in the aircraft world, if the plane is unsafe, you can get another one if needed. In the patient care world, that really isn't an option; you have to work for the patient who presents.

Even with the above differences taken into account, there is still much that we have learned from other industries to help us improve safety in medicine. Perhaps among the most important lesson, in my opinion, is that the concept of safety in surgery requires examining every aspect of every system and element that bears upon the patient outcome. None of us exists in isolation, and we are all interdependent on all of our other colleagues and facilities. It has been said that "success has a thousand fathers and failure is an orphan." I would posit that when we have a failure that our failure too has multiple parents, as it is usually an error chain that leads to truly bad outcomes.

In order to understand where and how we fit into a system of safety, we must first learn the vocabulary and tools that allow us to function more safely. Becoming facile with human factors, pathways, processes, and risk-mitigation as well as understanding the concepts of improving teamwork, analyzing data, and creating a culture that values safety, is critical to creating an environment that will minimize unnecessary bad outcomes. We are deeply indebted to Dr Zheng and her colleagues for compiling an excellent set of reviews that will allow the reader to develop a sound basis for continued education.

At the end of the day, those who work in our profession will not likely eliminate all bad outcomes. That said, we can do a great deal to create platforms that will allow us to minimize unnecessary risk. That journey to greater safety begins with a single step for all of us, and each of us needs to take that step; none of us can do this alone. It by definition requires a collective effort.

Looking back at the changes chronicled in *Surgical Clinics* series over the past 100 years, one may be struck by not just how much has changed but also by how much has stayed the same. We do live in an era with a sound foundation upon which we can build. We should neither feel as if we have made no progress nor should we feel complacent. We at *Surgical Clinics* greatly look forward to working with our readership and our contributors to generate the best and most useful information we can for the next century and more.

Ronald F. Martin, MD, FACS
Colonel (retired)
United States Army Reserve
York, Maine

E-mail address:
rfmcescna@gmail.com

Preface
Captain of the Ship

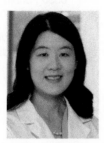

Feibi Zheng, MD, MBA, FACS
Editor

Over the course of my surgical training and as my practice has matured, I have come to realize that while technical excellence is a laudable goal, it is only 1 component of providing high-quality, cost-conscious, safe patient care. Surgery is becoming more complex with new technology, new data, and new organizational structures. While some may decry the loss of surgeon autonomy as our teams become increasingly multidisciplinary and diverse, we must recognize that our primary goal is to do what is best for the patient. Creating, adapting, and embracing these new frameworks for patient safety will enable us to provide higher-quality care. In this issue, we explore the evolution of these ideas and provide practical tools and frameworks for implementation at your local institution. In the first few articles, we acknowledge the importance of human factors in the design of surgical systems, the need for clear communication between members of the health care team, and how standardization can minimize harm. In the middle section, we examine how technology can help us identify patients at risk for adverse events and how technology can enable us to help patients recover safely at home. Finally, 3 articles examine how we can measure and track patient safety events, the cost of implementing patient safety programs balanced against the cost of patient harm, and how we train the next generation of surgeons in these principles. Surgeons remain the captain of the ship, but now we navigate increasingly choppy waters with a bigger crew and more complicated equipment. It is our hope that

Surg Clin N Am 101 (2021) xvii–xviii
https://doi.org/10.1016/j.suc.2020.09.013
0039-6109/21/© 2020 Published by Elsevier Inc.

surgical.theclinics.com

this issue provides you with ideas and tools to help you keep your patients safe and well in their surgical journey.

Feibi Zheng, MD, MBA, FACS
Houston Methodist Hospital
6550 Fannin Street
Houston, TX 77030, USA

E-mail address:
fzheng@houstonmethodist.org

A Human Factors Approach to Surgical Patient Safety

Tara N. Cohen, PhD[a], Bruce L. Gewertz, MD[a], Daniel Shouhed, MD[b],*

KEYWORDS

- Human factors • Surgery • Patient safety • SEIPS • Ergonomics

KEY POINTS

- Although errors can be attributed to individuals, they are often the product and natural consequences of defective systems that allow errors to go unnoticed.
- The operating room provides multiple opportunities for suboptimal communication, discordant motivations, and errors arising from cognitive biases, poor interpersonal skills, and substandard environmental factors; these are all independent of technical incompetence.
- "Human factors research" can be described as the study and design of environments and processes to ensure safer, more effective, and more efficient systems, thereby enhancing human performance.
- Human factors methods for *studying* patient safety in surgery include observational studies, retrospective review, and the use of surveys, interviews, and focus groups.
- Human factors methods for *improving* patient safety in surgery include the implementation of checklists, briefings, team training, handoff protocols, and interventions focused on well-being.

THE HISTORY AND EVOLUTION OF HUMAN FACTORS
What Is Human Factors?

The safety and well-being of patients within the hospital system is the fundamental mission of most institutions. That said, the imperfect nature of humans incorporates vulnerability within systems such that errors and adverse events are unavoidable. Many errors have little to no consequence and often go unnoticed; occasionally they translate into an important adverse event.

A growing consensus acknowledges that although errors and adverse events are often committed by individuals, they are mostly the product and natural consequences of defective systems and inadequate organizational structures that allow

[a] Department of Surgery, Cedars-Sinai Medical Center, 8700 Beverly Boulevard, North Tower, Suite 8215, Los Angeles, CA 90048, USA; [b] Department of Surgery, Cedars-Sinai Medical Center, 8635 West Third Street, West Medical Office Tower, Suite 650-W, Los Angeles, CA 90048, USA
* Corresponding author.
E-mail address: Daniel.Shouhed@cshs.org

Surg Clin N Am 101 (2021) 1–13
https://doi.org/10.1016/j.suc.2020.09.006
0039-6109/21/© 2020 Elsevier Inc. All rights reserved.

errors to go unnoticed.[1–4] Beyond their cost in human lives, preventable medical errors result in financial costs projected to be between $17 billion and $29 billion per year in US hospitals.[5]

Human factors can be described as the study and design of environments and processes within a system to ensure safer, more effective, and more efficient performance by humans.[6–9] Within the realm of health care, human factors engineers strive to maximize human performance and system efficiency, while promoting health, safety, comfort, and quality of life.[4,9,10] Errors represent the mental or physical activities of individuals that fail to achieve their intended outcome. They can be a result of poor decision making, inadequate skill, or inaccurate perception.[11] Errors can be intercepted by appropriate actions that can minimize threat to patient safety.[4] An adverse event is any unintended consequence of medical treatment that results in prolonged hospital stay, morbidity, or mortality. It may also be an injury caused by medical management rather than by the underlying condition of the patient.[8]

The "Swiss Cheese" model of accident causation provides a theoretic framework for the cause of errors within the context of systems. According to this model, accidents are a result of both active and latent failures. Active failures are unsafe acts committed by individuals at the frontline of the human-system interface whose actions can have immediate, adverse consequences. Latent failures are the result of poor systems design or decision making by members of the organizational and management staff. The long-term effects of latent failures may lie dormant for a period of time, only to surface when they combine with active failures. Each "slice of cheese" is analogous to a systemic defense against error, while the holes within each slice are a combination of active and latent failures. Occasionally, the holes within each layer of defense will perfectly line up together and allow an error to bypass the system's defenses, culminating into an accident or adverse event.[9,12]

Researchers have recognized the need for human factors engineering and have developed a model to empirically study system design as it relates to patient safety.[7] The Systems Engineering Initiative for Patient Safety (SEIPS) model is used widely in the field of human factors in medicine. According to this model, a *person* performs various *tasks* using different *tools and technologies* within a specific *physical environment* and under specific *organizational conditions*. The model places the individual at the center and carries the notion that all the elements of the system have an effect, not only on the individual but also on the other elements within the system. The SEIPS model suggests that surgical skill, overall performance, and outcomes are strongly affected by such factors as teamwork, communication, the physical working environment, technology, and other organizational variables.[7,9] For example, the introduction of a new technology, such as a surgical robot, requires new skills and tasks to be learned, a suitable environment in which to operate and maintain it, as well as economic and structural support provided by the organization.

The Evolution of Human Factors Outside of Medicine

Humans have often been concerned with identifying ways to improve performance in various aspects of work and daily life. In the late 1800s, around the time of the Industrial Revolution, there was a demand to increase the efficiency of humans in the workplace.[13] Fredrick Winslow Taylor is most famous for his shovel study conducted at the Bethlehem Steel Company. Taylor studied and modified the selection of workers, their training, and work-rest schedules to improve efficiency and output. He developed a series of shovels designed specifically for moving different types of materials, in contrast to the use of a single, universal tool. Ultimately, he was able to increase worker daily output from 12.5 to 47.5 tons per day.[13]

During World War II, advances in technology allowed for the development of new, complex machinery. Heightened complexity required higher cognitive demand by the operators. Among all accidents resulting in US Army Air Corps pilot losses during war time, two-thirds occurred as a result of training crashes and operational accidents.[14] The similarity between the insignia of US and Japanese aircraft led to US pilots tragically shooting down friendly planes. Engineers recognized the defective design and made changes to easily distinguish between friendly and enemy planes, significantly reducing self-inflicted casualties (**Fig. 1**).

The potential for accidental mass casualties within commercial aviation gave even more motivation to further the science of human factors. Over the last half-century, many changes have occurred to optimize crew resource management, equipment design, as well as procedural and organizational practices. Modifications in instrument display and control knob configuration have allowed for safer and more efficient use by pilots.[15] Closed-loop communication and the use of a universal language have facilitated the accurate delivery and understanding of information.[16–18] Indeed, human factors research within the aviation industry has provided an exemplary template for creating a system of safety within health care.

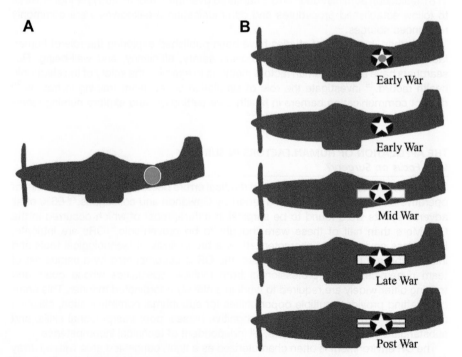

Fig. 1. Aircraft insignia changes. (*A*) Japanese Hinomaru National Air insignia. (*B*) United States National Air insignia changes over time.

The Evolution of Human Factors in Medicine and Surgery

Although human factors has been recognized as an essential field to improve safety and efficiency in several industries, it has been slower to enter health care professions. Given the complexity of health care, interventions that do not take into consideration all elements in a given system are not likely to successfully improve patient safety and quality of care.[19] Moreover, in a health care setting, unlike many others, a caregiver's successful performance will impact not only their own well-being but also the outcomes for another person, the patient.

Hippocrates was one of the first to formally make concrete recommendations for surgeons and their work environments to enhance performance. He discussed relative positioning of the surgeon and the patient, emphasizing the importance of ergonomic comfort while performing procedures. Hippocrates also stressed the importance of the location, size, and weight of instruments in addition to the layout of light sources.[20] Each of the factors identified by Hippocrates has become immensely important across surgery and even other types of performance.

Through use of video recording, engineers Frank and Lillian Gilbreth, would observe surgeons and analyze each of their movements to see if they could make their work more efficient and less fatiguing. They suggested the involvement of operating room (OR) nurses and the standardization of surgical instrument layout to improve efficiency.[21] During the mid-twentieth century, Safren and Chapanis[22–24] conducted one of the first studies of human factors and medication safety through the application of critical incident reporting to identify medication errors. They achieved this by collecting data on direct observations of human behavior and analyzing their effects. The investigators found that several types of work system factors contributed to the 178 medication administration errors captured over the 7-month study period. Failures to follow established procedures and communication breakdowns were commonly referenced sources.

Since then, hundreds of studies have been published exploring the role of human factors research in medicine for improving safety, efficiency, and well-being. Researchers have applied human factors methods to examine the safety of the electronic health record,[25] investigate the role of simulation-based team training in trauma,[26] dissect communication barriers in health care settings,[27] and explore nursing workload and its impact on patient safety.[28]

THE APPLICATION OF HUMAN FACTORS IN SURGERY
Why Focus on Surgery?

Surgery accounts for a large number of medical errors because of the critical nature of operative interventions. In fact, in a report by Gawande and colleagues,[29] 66% of all adverse events were found to be surgical in nature, most of which occurred in the OR. More than half of these were thought to be preventable.[9] ORs are intricate, high-stress environments characterized by a broad array of technological tools and interdisciplinary personnel. Furthermore, the OR is accompanied by a unique set of team dynamics, where professionals from multiple specialties whose goals and training differ widely are required to work in a closely coordinated manner. This complex setting provides multiple opportunities for suboptimal communication, clashing motivations, and errors arising from cognitive biases, poor interpersonal skills, and substandard environmental factors, all independent of technical incompetence.

The OR environment is often characterized as a tight, congested area with an array of wires, tubes, and lines, known as the "spaghetti syndrome."[30] Consequently, movements by members of the surgical team are often obstructed; instruments and supplies may be difficult to access and maintain, and the risk of accidental disconnection of devices and human error increases.[31] Poor lighting, suboptimal temperature, and excessive or unwanted noise have been shown to negatively affect surgical performance.[32] Unnecessary noise may also hinder appropriate communication needed among the OR staff.

Poor communication has been increasingly regarded as a causal factor in a large percentage of sentinel events within the health care system.[33] The Joint Commission reports communication as the number 1 root cause of sentinel events from 1995 through 2004. In 1 study, incomplete or erroneous communication was a causal factor in 43% of errors made during surgery.[34] The interplay between different members of the surgical team is yet another critical component of surgical performance. Studies have shown that teamwork factors alone account for 45% of the variance in errors committed by surgeons during cardiac cases.[35] The stability of a cohesive team fosters the development of trust among its members and allows for a smooth progression of the case. All would agree that improving the design of the surgical environment and equipment, the order, allocation, and definition of surgical tasks, and fostering the development of cohesive teams through excellent communication would naturally enhance surgical performance and outcomes.

Human Factors Methods of Studying Surgical Patient Safety

Observational studies

Human factors focuses on studying elements of an underlying system. Several methods have been developed to study unique processes in a variety of industries. In fact, Stanton and colleagues[36] discuss more than 100 methods in their textbook: "Human Factors Methods: A Practical Guide for Engineering and Design." Although many of the methods outlined by Stanton could be applied to surgery, the authors have selected a few of the most commonly used methods in the field.

One approach involves conducting detailed observations of the processes, people, and interactions that take place in a particular area. Observational research is simple yet can be very helpful for understanding how individuals in a given setting function in reality. Catchpole and colleagues[37] argue that direct observation of health care processes allow for the examination of how work is truly accomplished in a given environment (*work done*) in contrast to how individuals believe work should be completed within a system (*work imagined*). This type of research allows for the study of a variety of system-level factors, such as communication breakdowns, poor teamwork and coordination, issues with environmental workspace, technological failures, and challenges associated with organizational leadership and culture.

One common approach for studying the work system via observation is to collect flow disruptions or "deviations in the natural progression of an operation, thereby compromising the safety of an operation."[35] Flow disruptions include issues like impaired teamwork, communication breakdowns, extraneous interruptions, and equipment problems. Wiegmann and colleagues[35] were the first to formally study flow disruptions. Researchers observed 31 cardiac surgical procedures and demonstrated that surgical errors increase significantly with the increase of flow disruptions. Shouhed and colleagues[38] studied flow disruptions in trauma surgery. Over a 10-week period, researchers observed 87 cases and identified 1759 flow disruptions. Most of the flow disruptions identified in the OR were related to coordination issues and communication breakdowns. Investigators argued that flow disruptions can be used not only as a surrogate for efficiency and quality measures but also as a diagnostic tool for understanding systems-level problems in trauma care.[39]

In a 2016 study, researchers at Embry-Riddle Aeronautical University and the Medical University of South Carolina observed 15 cardiac surgery cases and identified 878 flow disruptions. Significant differences were identified in the frequency of flow disruptions experienced relative to the surgical team member discipline involved. For example, circulating nurses experienced more coordination and interruption-related disruptions than anesthesiologists and perfusionists, whereas anesthesiologists and perfusionists experienced a greater frequency of layout issues.[40]

Surveys, interviews, and focus groups

Although essential information about the underlying system can be discovered using observational research methods, observation is expensive and time-consuming and can be difficult to conduct reliably. Other commonly used human factors methods involve conducting surveys, interviews, and focus groups to evaluate team member perceptions of various elements in the system. Such methods can portray an accurate understanding of the current culture, teamwork environment, and even the usability of a newly introduced technology or process.

Surveys or questionnaires are convenient, anonymous, and cost-effective ways to assess the perceptions of individuals or groups in surgery. Today, several online platforms exist for conducting survey research that are secure and HIPAA compliant.[41] Makary and colleagues[42] developed the Safety Attitudes Questionnaire (SAQ), which measures 6 domains: teamwork climate, safety climate, job satisfaction, perceptions of management, stress recognition, and working conditions. Researchers later used the SAQ to study the impact of OR briefings on coordination of care and risk for wrong-site surgery. Results demonstrated that briefings were associated with caregiver perceptions of reduced risk for wrong-site surgery as well as improved collaboration.[43]

In another study, Cohen and colleagues[44] used a survey to investigate differences in perceptions surrounding robotic surgery turnover time. The investigators found that perceptions of contributors to lengthy turnover time varied by the type of team member surveyed. Surgeons and anesthesiologists thought that "time to set up the OR" was the greatest contributor to OR turnover, whereas circulating nurses and surgical technicians thought that "instrument availability" was the largest contributor to lengthy turnover times. Interestingly, the perceptions, or "work imagined," by both groups of participants was discordant with the objective observation that cleaning time was the longest component of OR turnover, once again stressing the value of direct observation. Relying solely on survey data may provide inaccurate information about the current state of a system based on the individual biases of participants; however, surveys provide insight into the current attitudes and cultures that exist within the institution. It is important to know what the perceptions are surrounding a given system before universal changes can be made.

Focus groups are another method used to understand users and their perceptions. Focus groups can be a powerful tool in system development and can be used to uncover what users truly want and need from a system.[45] In a 2007 study from Iceland, researchers conducted focus groups to identify threats to patient safety in the OR to discover how OR nurses can play an active role in ensuring safety. Results from the focus groups highlighted potential weaknesses in the system, such as the understaffing of teams resulting in the need to pull support from other teams.[46]

Retrospective review

Incident reports are an additional source of valuable information that may provide insights into the function of a health care system. When incidents are appropriately documented, "near misses" described in the reports provide valuable information to health care organizations regarding failures that may exist in the system. When evaluated, incident reports generate opportunities to mitigate systemic vulnerabilities before a patient harm event occurs.[47] Human factors approaches can be used to identify systemic vulnerabilities that exist in an incident report. In a 2018 study, researchers applied the Human Factors Analysis and Classification System for Healthcare (HFACS-Healthcare) to surgical near-miss events reported via a hospital's event reporting system over the course of 1 year. Within the 592 events analyzed, 726 contributing factors were identified. Most issues revolved around failures of the preconditions for unsafe acts tier of the HFACS-Healthcare framework, namely communication breakdowns, poor coordination, and workspace design issues.[48]

Unlike traditional incident reviews, simulation can be used to reconstruct accidents and scenarios to enhance the detection of error and adverse events. A 2014 study by Slakey and colleagues[49] developed and evaluated the use of simulation scenarios to investigate the causality of adverse surgical outcomes. Researchers reviewed 631 closed medical malpractice claims and selected 3 cases for simulation. Simulation scenarios were developed using abstracted data from the medical malpractice records, and sources of error were identified and compared between the simulations and the closed claims. More systemic errors were identified in the simulation of adverse outcomes compared with the closed claims. In addition, when compared with conventional root cause analysis, simulation of adverse outcomes identified more systems-based error rather than errors committed by individuals.

Human Factors Methods of Improving Surgical Patient Safety

Checklists
Once breakdowns in a work system have been identified, there are several approaches that can be used to improve patient safety. Perhaps one of the most commonly used interventions involves the use of a surgical checklist. Checklists can be useful when correctly used to reduce task demands placed on team members. They can ensure against errors of omission, promote explicit consistency of repetitive tasks, and improve procedural learning as well as process reliability.[12] Despite the efficacy of well-designed checklists, a poorly implemented one could itself lead to flow disruptions during the case. Thus, whereby such interventions do not complement existing systems of work, they may be met with cultural resistance, particularly when they are viewed as just a redundant task to complete.[50–52]

Haynes and colleagues[53] developed the Surgical Safety Checklist to reduce morbidity and mortality in a global population. Researchers found that implementation of the checklist was associated with reductions in the rate of death and complications in patients undergoing noncardiac surgery. During the same year, researchers in Amsterdam developed the SURgical Patient Safety System (SURPASS) checklist, a multidisciplinary checklist that covers the entire surgical pathway.[54] A separate study implemented the SURPASS checklist to increase standardization in the surgical pathway and improve surgical patient safety specifically related to antibiotic prophylaxis. Researchers included 772 surgical procedures in the study (369 prechecklist implementation and 403 postchecklist implementation) and found that the implementation of the checklist significantly improved compliance with hospital standards for antibiotic prophylaxis administration.[55]

Briefings and team training
Preoperative and postoperative briefings involve a gathering of all team members to either plan or discuss ways to improve processes. Briefings enhance team awareness

and knowledge through shared information, explicit confirmation, reminders, and education. They also help to identify potential problems or disruptions before they occur, encourage prompt decision making, and initiate the completion of tasks in a timely, organized manner.[56] Briefings have also been shown to significantly reduce the risk of wrong-site surgery.[43] They encourage collaboration among OR staff and other members of the team. Studies have shown briefings to reduce delays, communication failures, and disruptions in surgical flow and allow better identification of problems and knowledge gaps.[57,58] Despite the benefits briefings provide, they may be viewed negatively by some because of associated delays and the need to simultaneously assemble all members of the OR.

To improve poor or ineffective communication and coordination, health care leaders have implemented team training interventions. Several team training curriculums have been applied to enhance teamwork and communication in surgery, the most well-known being TeamSTEPPS. TeamSTEPPS, which stands for Team Strategies and Tools to Enhance Performance and Patient Safety, was developed by the Agency for Healthcare Research and Quality and the US Department of Defense. It is an evidence-based set of teamwork tools that aims to optimize patient outcomes by improving teamwork skills among health care professionals.[59,60] Teamwork training aims to improve interpersonal relationships through the improvement of nontechnical skills, such as communication and leadership. It has been shown to deliver better team skills, better satisfaction with care, improved compliance with briefings, and reduced error rates.[61–64] Team training can also lead to better organizational perceptions that help sustain institutional change.[65] Improved teamwork ultimately leads to intersecting goals among team members, thereby improving the flow with which an operation progresses.

Handoff protocols
Another area that may benefit from human factors involvement involves the handoff of patients between team members. Handoffs can occur within the same space between members of the same team (eg, when an anesthesiologist returns to the OR after taking a break) or between different teams from different locations (eg, when the patient is handed off from the OR team to the postanesthesia care unit team). Perioperative handoffs are particularly susceptible to error given the need to simultaneously manage the physical transfer of the patient while coordinating complex technology and transferring a large amount of critical information.

Breakdowns in communication among team members often occur during the handoff of patients from 1 team to another (eg, from the OR team to the intensive care unit [ICU] team). With an aim to improve safety and quality of patient handoff in a critical period, Catchpole and colleagues[66] developed a simple, reliable protocol to be used in the handoff between the surgical and ICU team after complex congenital heart surgery. The handoff protocol was developed following detailed discussions with a Formula 1 racing team and aviation training captains. Researchers observed 50 patients before and after implementation of the handoff protocol and collected data on technical errors, omission of information, and teamwork. The mean number of technical errors and handover omissions were significantly reduced following the implementation of the protocol.

Interventions focused on well-being
Factors associated with well-being can greatly impact surgical performance. Cognitive and physical stressors in the OR, like technical complications, distractions,

interruptions, time pressure, awkward positioning, and increased workload, can negatively impact technical and nontechnical skills.[9,67,68]

Physical well-being may be improved by addressing intraoperative ergonomic risk factors impacting surgeons.[69] In an effort to mitigate the ergonomic risks presented to surgeons in the OR, researchers studied the impact of incorporating surgical microbreaks (short breaks about 1 minute every 20–30 minutes) in surgery.[70] Researchers recruited 56 attending surgeons to participate in 1 day of regular surgeries and a second day of surgeries including microbreaks followed by questions. Surgeons reported improvement or no change in their mental focus and physical performance on the days that they completed the microbreaks. In addition, discomfort in the shoulders was significantly reduced. The surgical microbreaks did not cause significant distraction or disruption to the flow of the procedure, and 87% of the surgeons wanted to incorporate microbreaks into their OR routine.[70]

Institutions like the Mayo Clinic[71] and Stanford University[72] have implemented physician well-being and life balance programs that aim to provide physicians with resources and strategies for combating mental well-being challenges, such as burnout. Although both programs show promise for success, they are rare in surgery.[73]

SUMMARY

Despite increased awareness of safety, errors routinely continue to occur in surgical care. Disruptions in the flow of an operation, such as teamwork and communication failures, contribute significantly to adverse events. Although it is apparent that some incidence of human error is unavoidable, there is evidence in medicine and other fields that systems can be better designed to prevent or detect errors before a patient is harmed. The complexity of factors leading to surgical errors requires collaboration between surgeons and human factors experts to carry out the proper prospective and observational studies. Only when we are guided by this valid and real-world data can useful interventions be identified and implemented. Improving the design of equipment, the order, allocation, and definition of surgical tasks, the design of the surgical environment, and the organization of services and support around the maintenance and improvement of surgical flow could all yield improvements in surgical performance and eventually caregiver and patient outcomes.

CLINICS CARE POINTS

Pearls

- One of the best approaches to studying patient safety from a human factors perspective involves conducting observational research. Direct observation of healthcare processes allow for the examination of how work is truly accomplished in a given environment.
- Flow disruption research can be used as a surrogate for efficiency and quality measures as well as a diagnostic tool for understanding systems-level problems in healthcare.
- Surveys and questionnaires are convenient, anonymous and cost-effective ways to assess the perceptions of individuals or groups in surgery.
- When incidents are appropriately documented, "near misses", described in the reports provide valuable information to healthcare organizations regarding the failures that might contribute to patient safety.

Pitfalls

- Observational research is expensive, time consuming and can be difficult to conduct reliably

- Subjective measurement methods (e.g., surveys, interviews) provide insight into current perspectives of the individuals involved, but may not accurately reflect current processes.

DISCLOSURE

The authors have nothing to disclose.

REFERENCES

1. Ta B, Leape LL, Laird NM, et al. Incidence of adverse events and negligence in hospitalized patients. Results of the Harvard Medical Practice Study I. N Engl J Med 1991;324:370–6.
2. Homsted L. Institute of Medicine report: to err is human: building a safer health care system. Fla Nurse 2000;48(1):6.
3. de Vries EN, Ramrattan MA, Smorenburg SM, et al. The incidence and nature of in-hospital adverse events: a systematic review. BMJ Qual Saf 2008;17(3): 216–23.
4. Etchells E, O'Neill C, Bernstein M. Patient safety in surgery: error detection and prevention. World J Surg 2003;27(8):936–41.
5. Thomas EJ, Lipsitz SR, Studdert DM, et al. The reliability of medical record review for estimating adverse event rates. Ann Intern Med 2002;136(11):812–6.
6. Association IE. What is ergonomics. IEA. 2020. Available at: https://www.iea.cc/whats/index.html. Accessed September 1, 2019.
7. Carayon P, Hundt AS, Karsh BT, et al. Work system design for patient safety: the SEIPS model. BMJ Qual Saf 2006;15(suppl 1):i50–8.
8. Kohn LT, Corrigan J, Donaldson MS. To err is human: building a safer health system, vol. 6. Washington, DC: National academy press; 2000.
9. Shouhed D, Gewertz B, Wiegmann D, et al. Integrating human factors research and surgery: a review. Arch Surg 2012;147(12):1141–6.
10. Carayon P, Xie A, Kianfar S. Human factors and ergonomics as a patient safety practice. BMJ Qual Saf 2014;23(3):196–205.
11. Shappell SA, Wiegmann DA. The human factors analysis and classification system–HFACS. 2000.
12. Reason J. Human error. New York: Cambridge university press; 1990.
13. Meister D. The history of human factors and ergonomics. Boca Raton (FL): CRC Press; 2018.
14. Army Air Forces Washington DC Office of Statistical Control. Army Air Forces Statistical Digest (World War II) Accession Number: ADA542518. 1945:121.
15. Fitts PM, Jones RE. Psychological aspects of instrument display: analysis of 270" pilot error" experiences in reading and interpreting aircraft instruments (No. TSEAA-694-12A). Dayton, OH: Aeromedical Laboratory; 1947. Air Material Command.
16. Leape LL, Berwick DM, Bates DW. What practices will most improve safety?: evidence-based medicine meets patient safety. JAMA 2002;288(4):501–7.
17. Helmreich RL, Merritt AC, Wilhelm JA. The evolution of crew resource management training in commercial aviation. Int J Aviat Psychol 1999;9(1):19–32.
18. Salas E, Wilson KA, Murphy CE, et al. Communicating, coordinating, and cooperating when lives depend on it: tips for teamwork. Jt Comm J Qual Patient Saf 2008;34(6):333–41.
19. Carayon P, Wetterneck TB, Rivera-Rodriguez AJ, et al. Human factors systems approach to healthcare quality and patient safety. Appl Ergon 2014;45(1):14–25.

20. Marmaras N, Poulakakis G, Papakostopoulos V. Ergonomic design in ancient Greece. Appl Ergon 1999;30(4):361–8.
21. Baumgart A, Neuhauser DFrank and Lillian Gilbreth: scientific management in the operating room BMJ Quality & Safety 2009;18:413–415.
22. Flanagan JC. The critical incident technique. Psychol Bull 1954;51(4):327.
23. Safren MA, Chapanis A. A critical incident study of hospital medication errors. Nurs Res 1960;9(4):223.
24. Safren MA, Chapanis A. A critical incident study of hospital medication errors. Part 2. Hospitals 1960;34:53.
25. Sittig DF, Singh H. Eight rights of safe electronic health record use. JAMA 2009; 302(10):1111–3.
26. Weaver SJ, Salas E, Lyons R, et al. Simulation-based team training at the sharp end: a qualitative study of simulation-based team training design, implementation, and evaluation in healthcare. J Emerg Trauma Shock 2010;3(4):369.
27. Guttman OT, Lazzara EH, Keebler JR, et al. Dissecting communication barriers in healthcare: a path to enhancing communication resiliency, reliability, and patient safety. J Patient Saf 2018. https://doi.org/10.1097/PTS.0000000000000541.
28. Carayon P, Gurses AP. Nursing workload and patient safety—a human factors engineering perspective. In: Hughes RG, editor. Patient safety and quality: an evidence-based handbook for nurses. Rockville (MD): Agency for Healthcare Research and Quality (US); 2008. p. 203–13.
29. Gawande AA, Thomas EJ, Zinner MJ, et al. The incidence and nature of surgical adverse events in Colorado and Utah in 1992. Surgery 1999;126(1):66–75.
30. Brogmus G, Leone W, Butler L, et al. Best practices in OR suite layout and equipment choices to reduce slips, trips, and falls. AORN J 2007;86(3):384–98.
31. Ofek E, Pizov R, Bitterman N. From a radial operating theatre to a self-contained operating table. Anaesthesia 2006;61(6):548–52.
32. Healey AN, Sevdalis N, Vincent CA. Measuring intra-operative interference from distraction and interruption observed in the operating theatre. Ergonomics 2006; 49(5–6):589–604.
33. Carthey J, de Leval MR, Reason JT. The human factor in cardiac surgery: errors and near misses in a high technology medical domain. Ann Thorac Surg 2001; 72(1):300–5.
34. Gawande AA, Zinner MJ, Studdert DM, et al. Analysis of errors reported by surgeons at three teaching hospitals. Surgery 2003;133(6):614–21.
35. Wiegmann DA, ElBardissi AW, Dearani JA, et al. Disruptions in surgical flow and their relationship to surgical errors: an exploratory investigation. Surgery 2007; 142(5):658–65.
36. Stanton NA, Rafferty LA, Walker GH, et al. Human factors methods: a practical guide for engineering and design. 2nd ediiton. Boca Raton (FL): CRC Press; 2013.
37. Catchpole K, Neyens DM, Abernathy J, et al. Framework for direct observation of performance and safety in healthcare. BMJ Qual Saf 2017;26(12):1015.
38. Shouhed D, Blocker R, Gangi A, et al. Flow disruptions during trauma care. World J Surg 2014;38(2):314–21.
39. Blocker RC, Duff S, Wiegmann D, et al. Flow disruptions in trauma surgery: type, impact, and affect. 2012.
40. Cohen TN, Cabrera JS, Sisk OD, et al. Identifying workflow disruptions in the cardiovascular operating room. Anaesthesia 2016;71(8):948–54.

41. Harris PA, Taylor R, Thielke R, et al. Research electronic data capture (REDCap)—a metadata-driven methodology and workflow process for providing translational research informatics support. J Biomed Inform 2009;42(2):377–81.
42. Makary MA, Sexton JB, Freischlag JA, et al. Operating room teamwork among physicians and nurses: teamwork in the eye of the beholder. J Am Coll Surg 2006;202(5):746–52.
43. Makary MA, Mukherjee A, Sexton JB, et al. Operating room briefings and wrong-site surgery. J Am Coll Surg 2007;204(2):236–43.
44. Cohen TN, Anger JT, Shamash K, et al. Discovering the barriers to efficient robotic operating room turnover time: perceptions vs. reality. J Robot Surg 2020; 14(5):717–24.
45. Krueger RA. Focus groups: a practical guide for applied research. Thousand Oaks (CA): Sage publications; 2014.
46. Alfredsdottir H, Bjornsdottir K. Nursing and patient safety in the operating room. J Adv Nurs 2008;61(1):29–37.
47. Kaplan HS. Getting the right blood to the right patient: the contribution of near-miss event reporting and barrier analysis. Transfus Clin Biol 2005;12(5):380–4.
48. Cohen TN, Francis SE, Wiegmann DA, et al. Using HFACS-healthcare to identify systemic vulnerabilities during surgery. Am J Med Qual 2018;33(6):614–22.
49. Slakey DP, Simms ER, Rennie KV, et al. Using simulation to improve root cause analysis of adverse surgical outcomes. Int J Qual Health Care 2014;26(2):144–50.
50. Verdaasdonk EGG, Stassen LPS, Widhiasmara PP, et al. Requirements for the design and implementation of checklists for surgical processes. Surg Endosc 2009;23(4):715–26.
51. Manley R, Cuddeford JD. An assessment of the effectiveness of the revised FDA checklist. AANA J 1996;64(3):277–82.
52. Salvendy G. Handbook of human factors and ergonomics, vol. 144. New York: Wiley; 2006.
53. Haynes AB, Weiser TG, Berry WR, et al. A surgical safety checklist to reduce morbidity and mortality in a global population. N Engl J Med 2009;360(5):491–9.
54. de Vries EN, Hollmann MW, Smorenburg SM, et al. Development and validation of the SURgical PAtient Safety System (SURPASS) checklist. Qual Saf Health Care 2009;18(2):121–6.
55. de Vries EN, Dijkstra L, Smorenburg SM, et al. The SURgical PAtient Safety System (SUR-PASS) checklist optimizes timing of antibiotic prophylaxis. Patient Saf Surg 2010;4(1):6.
56. Lingard L, Regehr G, Orser B, et al. Evaluation of a preoperative checklist and team briefing among surgeons, nurses, and anesthesiologists to reduce failures in communication. Arch Surg 2008;143(1):12–7.
57. Henrickson SE, Wadhera RK, ElBardissi AW, et al. Development and pilot evaluation of a preoperative briefing protocol for cardiovascular surgery. J Am Coll Surg 2009;208(6):1115–23.
58. Nundy S, Mukherjee A, Sexton JB, et al. Impact of preoperative briefings on operating room delays: a preliminary report. Arch Surg 2008;143(11):1068–72.
59. Tibbs SM, Moss J. Promoting teamwork and surgical optimization: combining TeamSTEPPS with a specialty team protocol. AORN J 2014;100(5):477–88.
60. Weaver SJ, Rosen MA, DiazGranados D, et al. Does teamwork improve performance in the operating room? A multilevel evaluation. Jt Comm J Qual Patient Saf 2010;36(3):133–42.
61. Jankouskas T, Bush MC, Murray B, et al. Crisis resource management: evaluating outcomes of a multidisciplinary team. Simul Healthc 2007;2(2):96–101.

62. Halverson AL, Andersson JL, Anderson K, et al. Surgical team training: the North-western Memorial Hospital experience. Arch Surg 2009;144(2):107–12.
63. McCulloch P, Mishra A, Handa A, et al. The effects of aviation-style non-technical skills training on technical performance and outcome in the operating theatre. BMJ Qual Saf 2009;18(2):109–15.
64. Thomas EJ, Taggart B, Crandell S, et al. Teaching teamwork during the Neonatal Resuscitation Program: a randomized trial. J Perinatology 2007;27(7):409–14.
65. Morey JC, Simon R, Jay GD, et al. Error reduction and performance improvement in the emergency department through formal teamwork training: evaluation results of the MedTeams project. Health Serv Res 2002;37(6):1553–81.
66. Catchpole KR, De Leval MR, McEwan A, et al. Patient handover from surgery to intensive care: using Formula 1 pit-stop and aviation models to improve safety and quality. Pediatr Anesth 2007;17(5):470–8.
67. Hull L, Arora S, Kassab E, et al. Assessment of stress and teamwork in the operating room: an exploratory study. Am J Surg 2011;201(1):24–30.
68. Arora S, Sevdalis N, Nestel D, et al. The impact of stress on surgical performance: a systematic review of the literature. Surgery 2010;147(3):318–30.
69. Diller T, Helmrich G, Dunning S, et al. The human factors analysis classification system (HFACS) applied to health care. Am J Med Qual 2014;29(3):181–90.
70. Hallbeck MS, Lowndes BR, Bingener J, et al. The impact of intraoperative microbreaks with exercises on surgeons: a multi-center cohort study. Appl Ergon 2017;60:334–41.
71. Program on Physician Well-Being. Mayo Foundation for Medical Education and Research (MFMER). 2020. Available at: http://www.mayo.edu/research/centers-programs/physician-well-being-program/overview. Accessed February 24, 2020.
72. A Program to Create Balance in the Lives of our Residents. Stanford Medicine. 2020. Available at: http://med.stanford.edu/gensurg/education/BIL.html.
73. Dimou FM, Eckelbarger D, Riall TS. Surgeon burnout: a systematic review. J Am Coll Surg 2016;222(6):1230–9.

Teamwork and Surgical Team–Based Training

Akemi L. Kawaguchi, MD, MS[a],*, Lillian S. Kao, MD, MS[b]

KEYWORDS

- Surgery • Teamwork • Nontechnical skills • Simulation • Training

KEY POINTS

- Surgical teamwork is a critical component of safe and high-quality surgical care.
- Nontechnical skills can contribute to improvements in patient outcomes and operating room efficiency.
- Specific teamwork training programs exist and should be incorporated into surgical learning.

INTRODUCTION

Although surgical errors have historically been defined by the technical skill and clinical care of the surgeon, human factors often play a role in surgical complications. In a systematic review in 2008, DeVries found that 41% of in-hospital adverse events occurred in the operating room and 50% were related to an operation.[1] Factors such as teamwork failures—including breakdowns in communication, leadership, situational awareness, and conflict resolution—can contribute to both medical errors and patient harm.[2]

The operating room is a high-risk and time-sensitive environment. Thus, there is a strong need for excellent interdisciplinary communication and conflict management among surgical teams. Team members are diverse in their professional backgrounds and disciplines—including physicians, nurses, midlevel providers, students, and technicians from various specialties—and may only be together for a short period of time. The teams have a hierarchical structure, a high level of interdependence, high skill differentiation, and a sometimes high-stress environment.[3] In order to address these challenges, teamwork training for surgery has become a focus both in the workplace and as a part of surgical education.

[a] Department of Pediatric Surgery, McGovern Medical School at the University of Texas Health Science Center at Houston, 6431 Fannin Street, MSB 5.246, Houston, TX 77030, USA; [b] Division of Acute Care Surgery, Department of Surgery, McGovern Medical School at the University of Texas Health Science Center at Houston, 6431 Fannin Street, MSB 4.264, Houston, TX 77030, USA
* Corresponding author.
E-mail address: Akemi.Kawaguchi@uth.tmc.edu

Surg Clin N Am 101 (2021) 15–27
https://doi.org/10.1016/j.suc.2020.09.001
0039-6109/21/© 2020 Elsevier Inc. All rights reserved.

Surgical teamwork training borrows principles from aviation crew resource management, which can be defined as a family of instructional strategies that seek to improve teamwork in the cockpit by applying well-tested training tools and appropriate training methods targeted at specific content.[4] Crew resource management teamwork training for the operating room emphasizes nontechnical skills of the surgical team, rather than technical skills to perform the actual surgical procedure. These nontechnical skills are defined as the "cognitive and social skills that are not directly related to the surgeon's clinical knowledge, surgical dexterity, and technical performance."[5] Multiple studies have demonstrated that improvements in nontechnical skills such as communication and surgical teamwork can improve patient care, patient safety, operating room efficiency, and patient outcomes.[6–11]

In this article the authors review the definitions of teamwork attitude, teamwork behavior, nontechnical skills, and crew resource management. They also describe tools for assessing surgical teamwork, interventions to promote teamwork in a surgical setting, types and examples of teamwork training, and results of studies evaluating the association of teamwork with patient outcomes, both in and out of the operating room.

ASSESSMENT OF SURGICAL TEAMWORK

There are several tools that have been developed to assist with the measurement of both teamwork attitudes and behaviors. Teamwork attitudes are defined as the participant's perceptions of teamwork behaviors and the work environment, typically measured using validated questionnaires (**Table 1**). For example, the Teams Strategies and Tools to Enhance Performance and Patient Safety (TeamSTEPPS) Teamwork Attitudes Questionnaire (T-TAQ) is a tool that was developed by the Agency for Healthcare Research and Quality (AHRQ) to measure an individual's attitude toward core teamwork concepts, including team structure, leadership, situation monitoring, mutual support, and communication.[12,13] T-TAQ can be used to assess attitudes toward teamwork and the effectiveness of the TeamSTEPPS training program, which will be described in further detail later in the article. Other surveys measure teamwork attitudes as a component of safety culture—the shared beliefs, attitudes, values, norms, and behavioral characteristics of the staff attitudes and behaviors in relation to the organizational safety performance.[14] Safety culture as perceived by caregivers can be measured using several surveys (see **Table 1**), including the AHRQ Hospital Survey on Patient Safety Culture (SOPS), which assesses how providers and staff perceive various aspects of patient safety culture with composite measures on 10 components of patient safety, including 8 questions specifically about teamwork within and across units.[15] In addition, the Safety Attitudes Questionnaire (SAQ) is a validated and widely adopted tool that measures 6 domains of work environment and patient safety culture, assessing teamwork climate, the perceived quality of collaboration between personnel.[16]

Teamwork behaviors are observable, nontechnical actions that have been shown to contribute to performance in work environments such as health care.[8,17] Evaluation focuses on aspects of nontechnical skills, which include teamwork, communication, leadership, situational awareness, decision-making/problem solving, and conflict resolution. In order to evaluate the nontechnical skills of a surgical team, several validated tools evaluate teamwork and other nontechnical skills that contribute to team performance[18] (**Table 2**). These assessment tools can measure teamwork skills of multidisciplinary interprofessional or intraprofessional teams that include individuals within the same profession but at varied training levels.

Table 1 Assessment of teamwork attitudes		
Assessment Tool	**Measurement Scale**	**Teamwork Measurements**
Hospital Survey on Patient Safety AHRQ Survey (SOPS)[15]	5-point Likert	• In this unit, the authors work together as an effective team. • During busy times, staff in this unit help each other. • There is a problem with disrespectful behavior by those working in this unit.
Safety Attitudes Questionnaire (SAQ)[16]	5-point Likert	Teamwork climate • Nurse input is well received in this area • In this clinical area, it is difficult to speak up if a problem is perceived with patient care. • Disagreements in this clinical area are resolved appropriately (ie, not who is right, but what is best for the patient). • It is easy for personnel here to ask questions when there is something that they do not understand. • The physicians and nurses here work together as a well-coordinated team.
TeamSTEPPS Teamwork Attitudes Questionnaire (T-TAQ)[12]	5-point Likert	Six statements in 5 categories: • Team structure • Leadership • Situation monitoring • Mutual support • Communication

Data from Refs.[12,15,16]

Two validated measurement tools that are commonly used to evaluate *inter*disciplinary teamwork in the operating room.

Observational Teamwork Assessment for Surgery

Observational Teamwork Assessment for Surgery (OTAS) focuses on 5 teamwork elements, including communication, coordination/supportive behavior, collaboration, teamwork, and team monitoring/situational awareness. Exemplar behaviors are observed in 3 phases (preoperative, intraoperative, and postoperative) in either a simulated setting or during actual surgical cases. OTAS has been validated in many surgical subspecialties and languages.[19,20]

Revised Oxford Nontechnical Skills Scale

Revised Oxford Nontechnical Skills (NOTECHS) scale is adapted from an evaluation system used in the aviation industry, rating 4 behavioral dimensions—leadership and management, teamwork and cooperation, problem solving and decision-making, and situational awareness.[21] An adapted version of NOTECHS has also been used for the assessment of nontechnical skills during trauma resuscitation (T-NOTECHS)[22,23] and in various surgical subspecialties.[24,25]

Table 2
Assessment of nontechnical skills and teamwork behaviors

Name	Type of Team	Validated	Measurements of Teamwork Behaviors and Other NTS
Observational Teamwork Assessment in Surgery[19] (OTAS)	Interprofessional	Yes	Communication, coordination/supportive behavior, collaboration, teamwork, team monitoring/situational awareness in the preoperative, intraoperative, and postoperative phases
Oxford Nontechnical Skills System[21] (NOTECHS)	Interprofessional	Yes	Leadership & management, teamwork & cooperation, problem solving & decision-making, situation awareness
Nontechnical Skills for Surgeons (NOTSS)[27]	Intraprofessional	Yes	Situation awareness, decision-making, communication & teamwork, leadership
Surgeons' Leadership Inventory[32] (SLI)	Intraprofessional	No	Maintaining standards, managing resources, making decisions, directing, training, supporting others, communicating, coping with pressure
Anesthetists' Nontechnical Skills[34] (ANTS)	Intraprofessional	Yes	Task management, teamwork, situation awareness, decision-making
Scrub Practitioners' List of Intraoperative Nontechnical Skills[36] (SPLINTS)	Intraprofessional	Yes	Situation awareness, communication, and teamwork

Data from Refs.[19,21,27,32,34,36]

Three other tools assess *intra*professional nontechnical skills and teamwork within a particular profession in the operating room.

Nontechnical Skills of Surgeons

Nontechnical Skills of Surgeons (NOTSS) is a validated tool used to measure the nontechnical skills of surgeons in the operating room with evaluation of situation awareness, decision-making, communication and teamwork, and leadership.[17,26,27] This assessment tool has been used in a wide variety of surgical settings.[28–31]

Surgeon's Leadership Inventory

Surgeon's Leadership Inventory is used to assess the leadership skills of surgeons, including communicating, coping with pressure, maintaining standards, decision-making, managing resources, directing, training, and supporting others.[32,33]

Anesthetists' Nontechnical Skills

Anesthetists' Nontechnical Skills system examines behaviors in 15 elements, within 4 categories—task management, teamwork, situation awareness, and decision-making for anesthesiology teams.[34,35]

Scrub Practitioners' List of Intraoperative Nontechnical Skills

Scrub Practitioners' List of Intraoperative Nontechnical Skills is a tool used to evaluate the nontechnical skills of nurse and scrub technicians in situational awareness, communication, and teamwork.[36]

These assessments of teamwork attitudes and behaviors can be used to identify areas for improvement and evaluate the impact of teamwork interventions.

TEAMWORK INTERVENTIONS

Given the relationship between teamwork and nontechnical skills as well as patient and organizational outcomes, there have been numerous interventions studied to promote teamwork in a surgical setting. In a recent systematic review, Buljac-Samardzic and colleagues[37] described 3 types of teamwork interventions in health care: (1) training; (2) tools that structure, facilitate, or trigger teamwork (ie, checklists); and (3) organizational redesign to stimulate team processes and team functioning. In addition, programs have been developed that use a combination of these 3 types of interventions.[38,39] This review focuses on training tools and programs that have been used to improve surgical teamwork.

Teamwork Training

Principle-based training

Two commonly used types of principle-based teamwork training are crew resource management (CRM) and Teams Strategies and Tools to Enhance Performance and Patient Safety (TeamSTEPPS).

The National Aeronautics and Space Administration and aviation industry experts first developed CRM principles after evaluating the role of human error and nontechnical skills in flight safety.[4] In surgery, CRM is often used to teach nontechnical skills for the operating room.[11,40] Multiple studies have described the use of CRM training to enhance teamwork behaviors in the perioperative setting.

- In a 2019 systematic review of 64 articles on CRM in health care, Gross and colleagues noted that CRM interventions commonly included training on communication, situational awareness, leadership, teamwork, decision-making, briefing, error management, workload management, closed loop communication, and stress management. Effectiveness of CRM training can be evaluated with direct observation during simulation, learner evaluations and qualitative data, validated questionnaires, pre- and postintervention studies, and error or adverse outcome rates.[41]
- Tapson and colleagues combined CRM training, including principles related to teamwork, communication, and error avoidance, with venous thromboembolism prevention. The training resulted in immediate and retained confidence in identifying process-related factors leading to errors and improved compliance with venous thromboembolism prevention guidelines.[42]
- In a pre-/postintervention study of formal CRM training, McCulloch and colleagues used the SAQ and NOTECHS to evaluate teamwork attitude and behaviors. CRM training increased the mean SAQ mean teamwork score. Nontechnical teamwork skills also improved in the same time period. The mean overall technical errors also decrease following intervention.[43]

TeamSTEPPS, created by the United States Department of Defense and the AHRQ, is a widely used formal teamwork training program. TeamSTEPPS optimizes patient safety and quality of care by enhancing team structure and 4 teamwork competencies that include communication, leadership, situational monitoring, and mutual support.[44] The TeamSTEPPS training program consists of 3 phases: phase I—assessment, phase II—planning and implementation, and phase III—sustainment. Several studies have demonstrated an improvement in teamwork and clinical outcomes as well.

- In a TeamSTEPPS intervention on a Norwegian surgical ward, Aaberg and colleagues[45] found significantly improved scores in 3 SAQ safety culture dimensions including teamwork within unit and in 3 T-TAQ teamwork dimensions.
- In 2011, Forse and colleagues demonstrated a significant improvement in operating room teamwork and communication scores on the AHRQ Hospital SOPS, first case starts, and compliance with perioperative process measures, complications, and mortality. However, these changes were not sustained 1 year later.
- Pettker and colleagues implemented a comprehensive obstetric team training program using TeamSTEPPS and reported a significantly improved score for "a good teamwork climate" as assessed by the SAQ. Correspondingly, they also noted a decrease in Adverse Outcomes Index ($r^2 = 0.5$, $P = .01$) that included data for rates of both maternal and fetal outcomes.[46]

Despite these examples, there is a lack of consistent evidence for the effectiveness of TeamSTEPPS in improving nontechnical skills. In a scoping review of TeamSTEPPS in interprofessional education, Chen and colleagues found that some studies showed improved teamwork and communication with TeamSTEPPS training, but the outcomes were highly variable, potentially due to significant differences in implementation across educational contexts. Nonetheless, TeamSTEPPS training had an overall positive impact, is free, available online, and easily adaptable.[47]

Method-based training

Simulation-based training is a method-based training where appropriate teamwork processes can be instigated and by which team effectiveness can be measured and improved.[48] Using simulation, surgical trainees can acquire both technical and nontechnical skills without submitting patients to additional risk. More recently, simulation training has also been used to teach nontechnical skills including teamwork to surgical teams.

- Pucher and colleagues randomized groups of junior surgical residents to a half-day simulation training versus no training. Both groups then were observed during simulated ward rounds. The intervention group had significantly higher NOTECH scores for nontechnical skills and teamwork.[49]
- In a pre-/postintervention study, Rao and colleagues exposed 15 general surgery residents to a porcine gastrojejunostomy simulation and then had them perform 3 tasks that were designed to teach teamwork-related skills. The residents had significantly improved overall NOTSS scores with increased teamwork, leadership, and decision-making scores.[31]

In a review of 69 studies on simulation-based training, all reported improvements in some nontechnical skills and some reported improvements in technical skills. However, only a small percentage of these studies were of moderate to high quality.[37]

Tools for Teaching Teamwork

Teamwork tools are instruments that can be implemented to structure, facilitate, or trigger teamwork. Such tools can include checklists, rounding tools, structured debriefing,[43,50–54] and other communication techniques. The most widely used tool used to trigger teamwork behaviors and attitudes is the surgical safety checklists and debriefing, adapted from recommendations from the World Health Organization (WHO).[55–59] Haynes and colleagues[57] demonstrated significant improvements in morbidity and mortality after implementation of the checklist in 8 hospitals around the world, primarily associated with positive changes in teamwork and safety climate.[50] Briefings and debriefings are also often used after teamwork training as a time for team self-reflection and to give feedback about recently trained skills.[41,51,60–63]

Programmatic Teamwork Training

Programmatic training for teamwork combines multiple techniques, such as CRM combined with aspects of TeamSTEPPS, simulation, didactics, and tools. Programmatic training should also incorporate organizational context into program, making choices tailored to the needs of the local conditions. Numerous training programs that combine nontechnical skills and teamwork training have been developed and incorporated into surgical residency programs in the United States. Some examples, specifically for surgical residency training, are detailed in the following section.

- For general surgery training programs, the American College of Surgeons and the Association of Program Directors in Surgery (ACS/APDS) jointly developed a Resident Skills Curriculum, which includes simulation training modules with faculty moderators for nontechnical skills and teamwork competencies.[52] The course is freely available to members of the American College of Surgeons online, but costs and the extensive time commitment from both residents and faculty have been barriers to widespread implementation.[53,54,64] Rao and colleagues used scenarios from the ACS/APDS training program for 53 surgery, anesthesia, and nursing participants. Nontechnical skills were measured with the NOTECHS rating system, with all teams improving their scores from the first to the second scenario.[65]
- Dedy and colleagues performed a randomized controlled trial for junior surgical residents: conventional training versus nontechnical skill training intervention group. The intervention group outperformed their conventionally trained peers in knowledge of nontechnical skills, their attitudes toward teamwork as a means to improve patient safety, and their nontechnical performance during observed crisis simulations.[66]

In addition, programmatic teamwork training has also been used for multidisciplinary teams of professionals at various training levels.

- NetworkZ is a national, multidisciplinary team training program in New Zealand that focuses on improving patient safety by enhancing communication and teamwork in the operating room with high-fidelity simulation and specific instruction in communication strategies and speaking up and structured recaps. The NetworkZ program was originally run centrally and then transitioned over to one of the 20 local district health boards in New Zealand with central support. They noted that although they were able to show improvements in teamwork, this nationwide program required extensive organizational change and sustained support from hospital and the medical governing board of New Zealand.[67–69]
- In the United States Navy, the Surgical Trauma Training Course S2T2 is a 6-day mass casualty training program that emphasizes team dynamics to improve the delivery of multidisciplinary trauma care. The course begins with a didactic and

skills portion, then culminates in a full-day simulated mass casualty event with multiple waves of patients. When pre-/postprogram technical and nontechnical skills were assessed, all types of participants showed significant improvement.[56]

- Arriaga and colleagues developed a standardized operating room teamwork training curriculum that included principles of communication, assertiveness, and use of the WHO Surgical Safety Checklist. The course was delivered to 221 operating room staff from 4 hospitals at a central high-fidelity simulation center. The program was well received with 92.6% of the participants reporting that the training would help them provide safer patient care, with improvement in communication and assertiveness.[70]

Teamwork training is an effective means of improving teamwork skills to a wide variety of participants. The individual training assessment and training techniques can be customized to the needs and resources of individual programs and institutions.

RELATIONSHIP BETWEEN TEAMWORK AND PATIENT OUTCOMES

The ultimate goal for improving teamwork skills in surgical groups is to decrease errors and improve patient outcomes. Multiple observational studies have demonstrated a correlation between teamwork attitudes (ie, as reflected by safety culture) and surgical outcomes.

- In 2011, Haynes and colleagues implemented the WHO Safe Surgery Saves Lives checklist-based quality improvement project at 7 hospitals and found a significant increase in the mean teamwork and safety climate scores on the SAQ survey of operating room personnel. The rates of complications as assessed by parameters from the American College of Surgeons National Surgical Quality Improvement Program (NSQIP) decreased from a baseline of 11% to 7% following implementation.[50]
- In a study of general and vascular surgery teams from academic and Veterans Affairs hospitals, Davenport and colleagues administered the SAQ and a survey on perceived levels of communication and collaboration with coworkers. They correlated the risk-adjusted morbidity and mortality as assessed by the NSQIP with survey outcomes and determined that the reported communication and collaboration with attending and resident doctors correlated with risk-adjusted morbidity.[71,72]

Teamwork behaviors, of both individuals and teams, have also been correlated with surgical outcomes.

- Mishra and colleagues found that technical errors during 26 laparoscopic cholecystectomies as measured by the NOTECHS observation tool were negatively correlated with the surgeon's situational awareness scores ($\rho = .072$, $P<.001$). In addition, analysis of the correlation of SAQ score and outcomes showed a strong negative correlation between team situational awareness and technical errors.[10]
- Mazzocco and colleagues[8] demonstrated that patients who were cared for by surgical teams that exhibited good teamwork behaviors were less likely to experience major complications or death, even after adjusting for American Society of Anesthesiologists risk category.
- After implementing the Team STEPPS program, Forse and colleagues[44] reported a decrease in mortality from 2.7% to 1% ($P<.05$) and a reduction in overall surgical morbidity from 20.2% to 11% ($P<.05$).

SUMMARY

Effective teamwork is an essential component of safe and efficient surgical performance. Despite increasing recognition of the importance of teamwork and other nontechnical skills, most surgical training programs in the United States lack formalized, structured training. Several factors should be considered in determining the ideal teamwork training strategy for each institution. First, the type of teamwork training needs to be both effective and efficient, as time is very limited for both instructors and trainees. Second, cost and resources such as equipment and facilities must also be considered; thus, practice-based training using high-fidelity simulation may not be feasible in all contexts. Finally, a training program needs to have the support of leadership, with a significant investment of faculty, trainers, and financial backing. Although optimal timing and length of training not known, repetition and continued reinforcement are necessary to maintain teamwork skills. Teamwork training should be incorporated into several stages of medical school and residency training so that teamwork skills and attitude become a normal part of the surgical culture.

CLINICS CARE POINTS

- Effective surgical teamwork is an important component of patient care.
- Both technical and non-technical skills are essential parts of surgical training.

DISCLOSURE

The authors have no relevant conflicts of interest to disclose.

REFERENCES

1. De Vries EN, Ramrattan MA, Smorenburg SM, et al. The incidence and nature of in-hospital adverse events: a systematic review. Qual Saf Health Care 2008;17(3): 216–23.
2. Chung KC, Kotsis SV. Complications in surgery: root cause analysis and preventive measures. Plast Reconstr Surg 2012;129(6):1421–7.
3. Hollenbeck JR, Beersma B, Schouten ME. Beyond team types and taxonomies: a dimensional scaling conceptualization for team description. Acad Manage Rev 2012;37(1):82–106.
4. Salas E, Prince C, Bowers CA, et al. A methodology for enhancing crew resource management training. Hum Factors 1999;41(1):161–72.
5. Yule S, Flin R, Paterson-Brown S, et al. Non-technical skills for surgeons in the operating room: a review of the literature. Surgery 2006;139(2):140–9.
6. Greenberg CC, Regenbogen SE, Studdert DM, et al. Patterns of communication breakdowns resulting in injury to surgical patients. J Am Coll Surg 2007;204(4): 533–40.
7. Hull L, Arora S, Aggarwal R, et al. The impact of nontechnical skills on technical performance in surgery: a systematic review. J Am Coll Surg 2012;214(2): 214–30.
8. Mazzocco K, Petitti DB, Fong KT, et al. Surgical team behaviors and patient outcomes. Am J Surg 2009;197(5):678–85.
9. Dedy NJ, Fecso AB, Szasz P, et al. Implementation of an effective strategy for teaching nontechnical skills in the operating room. A single-blinded nonrandomized trial. Ann Surg 2016;263(5):937–41.

10. Mishra A, Catchpole K, Dale T, et al. The influence of non-technical performance on technical outcome in laparoscopic cholecystectomy. Surg Endosc 2008;22(1): 68–73.
11. Flin R, Maran N. Basic concepts for crew resource management and non-technical skills. Best Pract Res Clin Anaesthesiol 2015;29(1):27–39.
12. Baker DP, Amodeo AM, Krokos KJ, et al. Assessing teamwork attitudes in health-care: development of the TeamSTEPPS teamwork attitudes questionnaire. Qual Saf Health Care 2010;19(6):1–4.
13. Ballangrud R, Husebø SE, Hall-Lord ML. Cross-cultural validation and psycho-metric testing of the Norwegian version of TeamSTEPPS teamwork attitude ques-tionnaire. J Interprof Care 2020;34(1):116–23.
14. Morello RT, Lowthian JA, Barker AL, et al. Strategies for improving patient safety culture in hospitals: a systematic review. BMJ Qual Saf 2013;22(1):11–8.
15. Sorra JS, Dyer N. Multilevel psychometric properties of the AHRQ hospital survey on patient safety culture. BMC Health Serv Res 2010;10:199.
16. Sexton JB, Helmreich RL, Neilands TB, et al. The safety attitudes questionnaire: psychometric properties, benchmarking data, and emerging research. BMC Health Serv Res 2006;6:44.
17. Aveling EL, Stone J, Sundt T, et al. Factors influencing team behaviors in surgery: a qualitative study to inform teamwork interventions. Ann Thorac Surg 2018; 106(1):115–20.
18. Sharma B, Mishra A, Aggarwal R, et al. Non-technical skills assessment in sur-gery. Surg Oncol 2011;20(3):169–77.
19. Passauer-Baierl S, Hull L, Miskovic D, et al. Re-validating the observational team-work assessment for surgery tool (OTAS-D): cultural adaptation, refinement, and psychometric evaluation. World J Surg 2014;38(2):305–13.
20. Hull L, Bicknell C, Patel K, et al. Content validation and evaluation of an endovas-cular teamwork assessment tool. Eur J Vasc Endovasc Surg 2016;52(1):11–20.
21. Amaya Arias AC, Barajas R, Eslava-Schmalbach JH, et al. Translation, cultural adaptation and content re-validation of the observational teamwork assessment for surgery tool. Int J Surg 2014;12(12):1390–402.
22. Wieck MM, McLaughlin C, Chang TP, et al. Self-assessment of team performance using T-NOTECHS in simulated pediatric trauma resuscitation is not consistent with expert assessment. Am J Surg 2018;216(3):630–5.
23. Steinemann S, Berg B, Skinner A, et al. In situ, multidisciplinary, simulation-based teamwork training improves early trauma care. J Surg Educ 2011;68(6):472–7.
24. Saleh GM, Wawrzynski JR, Saha K, et al. Feasibility of human factors immersive simulation training in ophthalmology the london pilot. JAMA Ophthalmol 2016; 139(8):905–11.
25. Morgan L, Hadi M, Pickering S, et al. The effect of teamwork training on team per-formance and clinical outcome in elective orthopaedic surgery: A controlled inter-rupted time series study. BMJ Open 2015;5(4):e006216.
26. Jung JJ, Borkhoff CM, Jüni P, et al. Non-technical skills for surgeons (NOTSS): critical appraisal of its measurement properties. Am J Surg 2018;216(5):990–7.
27. Yule S, Gupta A, Gazarian D, et al. Construct and criterion validity testing of the non-technical skills for surgeons (NOTSS) behaviour assessment tool using videos of simulated operations. Br J Surg 2018;105(6):719–27.
28. Tsuburaya A, Soma T, Yoshikawa T, et al. Introduction of the non-technical skills for surgeons (NOTSS) system in a Japanese cancer center. Surg Today 2016; 46(12):1451–5.

29. Doumouras AG, Hamidi M, Lung K, et al. Non-technical skills of surgeons and anaesthetists in simulated operating theatre crises. Br J Surg 2017;104(8): 1028–36.
30. Yule S, Parker SH, Wilkinson J, et al. Coaching non-technical skills improves surgical residents' performance in a simulated operating room. J Surg Educ 2015; 72(6):1124–30.
31. Rao R, Dumon KR, Neylan CJ, et al. Can simulated team tasks be used to improve nontechnical skills in the operating room? J Surg Educ 2016;73(6): e42–7.
32. Parker SH, Flin R, McKinley A, et al. The surgeons' leadership inventory (SLI): a taxonomy and rating system for surgeons' intraoperative leadership skills. Am J Surg 2013;205(6):745–51.
33. Hu YY, Parker SH, Lipsitz SR, et al. Surgeons' leadership styles and team behavior in the operating room abstract presented at the American college of surgeons 101st annual clinical congress, scientific forum, Chicago, IL, October 2015. J Am Coll Surg 2016;222(1):41–51.
34. Fletcher G, Flin R, McGeorge M, et al. Anaesthetists' non-technical skills (ANTS): evaluation of a behavioural marker system. Br J Anaesth 2003;90(5):580–8.
35. Flin R, Patey R. Non-technical skills for anaesthetists: developing and applying ANTS. Best Pract Res Clin Anaesthesiol 2011;25(2):215–27. https://doi.org/10. 1016/j.bpa.2011.02.005.
36. Mitchell L, Flin R, Yule S, et al. Development of a behavioural marker system for scrub practitioners' non-technical skills (SPLINTS system). J Eval Clin Pract 2013; 192(2):317–23.
37. Buljac-Samardzic M, Doekhie KD, Van Wijngaarden JDH. Interventions to improve team effectiveness within health care: a systematic review of the past decade. Hum Resour Health 2020;18(1):1–42.
38. Hull L, Sevdalis N. Advances in teaching and assessing nontechnical skills. Surg Clin North Am 2015;95(4):869–84.
39. Stefanidis D, Sevdalis N, Paige J, et al. Simulation in surgery: what's needed next? Ann Surg 2015;261(5):846–53.
40. Wakeman D, Langham MR. Creating a safer operating room: groups, team dynamics and crew resource management principles. Semin Pediatr Surg 2018; 27(2):107–13.
41. Gross B, Rusin L, Kiesewetter J, et al. Crew resource management training in healthcare: a systematic review of intervention design, training conditions and evaluation. BMJ Open 2019;9(2):e025247.
42. Tapson VF, Karcher RB, Weeks R. Crew resource management and VTE prophylaxis in surgery: a quality improvement initiative. Am J Med Qual 2011;26(6): 423–32.
43. McCulloch P, Mishra A, Handa A, et al. The effects of aviation-style non-technical skills training on technical performance and outcome in the operating theatre. Qual Saf Health Care 2009;18(2):109–15.
44. Forse RA, Bramble JD, McQuillan R. Team training can improve operating room performance. Surgery 2011;150(4):771–8.
45. Aaberg OR, Hall-Lord ML, Husebø SIE, et al. A complex teamwork intervention in a surgical ward in Norway. BMC Res Notes 2019;12(1):1–7.
46. Pettker CM, Thung SF, Norwitz ER, et al. Impact of a comprehensive patient safety strategy on obstetric adverse events. Am J Obstet Gynecol 2009;200(5): 492.e1–8.

47. Chen AS, Yau B, Revere L, et al. Implementation , evaluation , and outcome of TeamSTEPPS in interprofessional education : a scoping review education : a scoping review. J Interprof Care 2019;33(6):795–804.
48. Gardner AK, Scott DJ. Concepts for developing expert surgical teams using simulation. Surg Clin North Am 2015;95(4):717–28.
49. Pucher PH, Aggarwal R, Singh P, et al. Ward simulation to improve surgical ward round performance: a randomized controlled trial of a simulation-based curriculum. Ann Surg 2014;260(2):236–43.
50. Haynes AB, Weiser TG, Berry WR, et al. Changes in safety attitude and relationship to decreased postoperative morbidity and mortality following implementation of a checklist-based surgical safety intervention. BMJ Qual Saf 2011;20(1):102–7.
51. Hicks CW, Rosen M, Hobson DB, et al. Improving safety and quality of care with enhanced teamwork through operating room briefings. JAMA Surg 2014;149(8):863–8.
52. American College of Surgeons. ACS/APDS surgery resident skills curriculum - phase 3. ACS/APDS Surgery Resident Skills Curriculum. Available at: https://learning.facs.org/content/acsapds-surgery-resident-skills-curriculum-phase-3. Accessed October 21, 2020.
53. Danzer E, Dumon K, Kolb G, et al. What is the cost associated with the implementation and maintenance of an ACS/APDS-based surgical skills curriculum? J Surg Educ 2011;68:519–25.
54. Pentiak PA, Schuch-Miller D, Streetman RT, et al. Barriers to adoption of the surgical resident skills curriculum of the American college of surgeons/association of program directors in surgery. Surgery 2013;154(1):23–8.
55. Hellar A, Tibyehabwa L, Ernest E, et al. A team-based approach to introduce and sustain the use of the WHO surgical safety checklist in Tanzania. World J Surg 2019;44(3):689–95.
56. Russ S, Rout S, Sevdalis N, et al. Do safety checklists improve teamwork and communication in the operating room? A systematic review. Ann Surg 2013;258(6):856–71.
57. Haynes AB, Weiser TG, Berry WR, et al. A surgical safety checklist to reduce morbidity and mortality in a global population. N Engl J Med 2009;360(5):491–9.
58. Singer SJ, Molina G, Li Z, et al. Relationship between operating room teamwork, contextual factors, and safety checklist performance. J Am Coll Surg 2016;223:568–80.
59. Erestam S, Haglind E, Bock D, et al. Changes in safety climate and teamwork in the operating room after implementation of a revised WHO checklist: a prospective interventional study. Patient Saf Surg 2017;11(1):4.
60. Gjeraa K, Spanager L, Konge L, et al. Non-technical skills in minimally invasive surgery teams: a systematic review. Surg Endosc 2016;30(12):5185–99.
61. Sundar E, Sundar S, Pawlowski J, et al. Crew resource management and team training. Anesthesiol Clin 2007;25(2):283–300.
62. Paige JT, Kozmenko V, Yang T, et al. High-fidelity, simulation-based, interdisciplinary operating room team training at the point of care. Surgery 2009;145(2):138–46.
63. Einav Y, Gopher D, Kara I, et al. Preoperative briefing in the operating room: shared cognition, teamwork, and patient safety. Chest 2010;137(2):443–9.
64. Korndorffer JR, Arora S, Sevdalis N, et al. The American college of surgeons/association of program directors in surgery national skills curriculum: adoption rate,

challenges and strategies for effective implementation into surgical residency programs. Surgery 2013;154(1):13–20.
65. Rao R, Caskey RC, Owei L, et al. Curriculum using the in-situ operating room setting. J Surg Educ 2017;74(6):e39–44.
66. Dedy NJ, Bonrath EM, Ahmed N, et al. Structured training to improve nontechnical performance of junior surgical residents in the operating room: A randomized controlled trial. Ann Surg 2016;263(1):43–9.
67. Jowsey T, Beaver P, Long J, et al. Towards a safer culture: implementing multidisciplinary simulation-based team training in New Zealand operating theatres - a framework analysis. BMJ Open 2019;9(10):e027122.
68. Weller J, Long JA, Beaver P, et al. Evaluation of the effect of multidisciplinary simulation-based team training on patients, staff and organisations: Protocol for a stepped-wedge cluster-mixed methods study of a national, insurer-funded initiative for surgical teams in New Zealand public h. BMJ Open 2020;10(2):1–8.
69. Weller J, Cumin D, Torrie J, et al. Multidisciplinary operating room simulation-based team training to reduce treatment errors: a feasibility study in New Zealand Hospitals. N Z Med J 2015;128(1418):40–51.
70. Arriaga AF, Gawande AA, Raemer DB, et al. Pilot testing of a model for insurer-driven, large-scale multicenter simulation training for operating room teams. Ann Surg 2014;259(3):403–10.
71. Davenport DL, Henderson WG, Mosca CL, et al. Risk-adjusted morbidity in teaching hospitals correlates with reported levels of communication and collaboration on surgical teams but not with scale measures of teamwork climate, safety climate, or working conditions. J Am Coll Surg 2007;205(6):778–84.
72. Awad SS, Fagan SP, Bellows C, et al. Bridging the communication gap in the operating room with medical team training. Am J Surg 2005;190(5):770–4.

Processes to Create a Culture of Surgical Patient Safety

Claire B. Rosen, MD[a],*, Rachel R. Kelz, MD, MSCE, MBA[b,c]

KEYWORDS

- Culture • Safety • Organization • Measurement • Education

KEY POINTS

- Creating a culture of patient safety starts at the top and requires substantial investment of time and resources.
- Teamwork and communication are paramount to establishing, changing, and continuing positive safety culture.
- Measurement is important not just for defining current culture but for identifying areas to enact change.
- There is national focus on the educational importance of patient safety, and a culture of patient safety, which should also be a focus of individual hospitals and training programs.

INTRODUCTION

Transforming the concepts of patient safety into a set of shared attitudes, values, goals, and practices that characterize an institution or organization must begin at the top and envelop each member of the organization. A culture of surgical safety requires devotion of the leadership to the safety mission, including dedicated time, focus, and financial investment.[1–3] Improved surgical patient safety and teamwork climate has been shown to improve patient outcomes, including surgical site infections and patient length of stay, so it is within the best interest of the organization to make safety a priority.[4,5] In addition, improved patient safety culture in itself is associated with better patient outcomes, improved efficiency, and fewer adverse events.[6–8] As such, the Joint Commission on Accreditation of Healthcare Organizations, the Institutes of Medicine, and the American College of Surgeons have each identified patient safety and the requisite culture of safety as a national focus.[1,9–11]

[a] Department of Surgery, Division of Surgical Education, Center for Surgery and Health Economics, Hospital of the University of Pennsylvania, 3400 Spruce Street, 4 Maloney, Philadelphia, PA 19104, USA; [b] Department of Surgery, Division of Endocrine and Oncologic Surgery, Center for Surgery and Health Economics, Hospital of the University of Pennsylvania, 3400 Spruce Street, 4 Silverstein, Philadelphia, PA 19104, USA; [c] University of Pennsylvania Perelman School of Medicine, Philadelphia, PA, USA
* Corresponding author.
E-mail address: claire.rosen@pennmedicine.upenn.edu

Surg Clin N Am 101 (2021) 29–36
https://doi.org/10.1016/j.suc.2020.09.008
0039-6109/21/© 2020 Elsevier Inc. All rights reserved.

surgical.theclinics.com

Although it may be difficult to identify and define specific actions that can create a culture of surgical patient safety, culture can be shaped through effort and action by the organization itself and through key interventions to be outlined in this article.

DISCUSSION

The investment of finances and focus in organizational infrastructure to support patient (and provider) safety must be visible to all stakeholders, including executive officers, organizational officers, and even board members, and must extend to all members of the organization and its patients. To enact any form of sustainable change, *resources* are needed, and the appropriate people to allow investment are those in control of the finances of the operation. Beyond the organizational leadership, there should be a committee on patient safety and advisory boards, which include supervisors, middle managers, risk managers, safety officers, quality improvement officers, physician staff, nursing staff, and other clinical staff.[12,13] This committee must make an active effort to focus not only on patient safety and quality improvement but also on the culture of the hospital or health care system with regard to patient safety as a whole. Furthermore, legal counsel of the health care system should be aligned to focus on patient safety agenda and appropriate accountability.[14]

Within each level of the system, it is important to create a "champion" or someone who can act as a role model and guide peer-to-peer conversations.[15,16] People are more receptive to feedback and more willing to enact change if they are hearing it from someone whom they trust and to whom they can relate. A risk manager telling nursing staff to feel comfortable speaking up in the operating room (OR) if they are concerned about a patient's safety is less meaningful than another nurse describing how he/she has handled similar situations in the past and the (hopefully) positive outcomes thereof. That being said, both managerial and staff perspectives are important when considering a change in culture, as both offer different insights into processes (one more subjective and based in emotion and existing culture and the other being more objective and able to identify gaps).[17] Another simple tool that can be invoked is the idea of executive walk rounds by more senior managerial members.[7] Even this simple exposure to leadership has been shown to be associated with better safety culture.[18,19]

Communication among stakeholders is critical to the establishment and maintenance of a culture of safety.[20,21] This holds true at all levels: surgeons must be able to speak freely with other surgeons, nursing, and clinical staff; nursing staff must be able to speak with organizational management; risk management must be able to speak with leaders and with nursing, etc. Patients and caregivers should be involved in open communication. Multidisciplinary staff should be united in regular meetings to discuss patient safety issues.[22] Teamwork should be a focus of health care systems and of surgical departments, with associated training on effective teamwork.[23,24] Storytelling should be encouraged and given meaningful attention from multiple levels. A focus of the system on open communication about patient safety is important to shaping the culture. **Table 1** organizes actions to promote a culture of safety by organizational tier.

In 2012, the American College of Graduate Medical Education (ACGME) launched a Clinical Learning Environment Review (CLER), in order to provide feedback to teaching hospitals on how well they engage residents with regard to patient safety and quality improvement.[25] These data then spurred the Pursuing Excellence Initiative (PEI) in 2015, which created a supportive network to share experiences and work together to create the best possible solutions in 6 areas of focus: patient safety, professionalism,

Table 1 Actions to promote a culture of safety by organizational tier	
Executives	• Identify and empower leaders of quality and safety (in surgery) • Invest in systems to generate and analyze clinical care • Recruit and hire data scientists and analysts • Access to measurement questionnaires • Walk rounds
Managers	• Serve as role models for quality and safety initiatives • Individualize programs • Incentivize participation in measurement questionnaires • Shift from "blame culture"
Surgeons/Physicians	• Champions within surgery • Mentorship • Lead safety process such as time-out and briefings • Set the tone of the OR • Record, report, and review all events and near misses (event reporting systems)
Nursing	• Use narrative medicine to encourage others to speak up/storytelling • Participation in measurement questionnaires • Event reporting systems • Participate and model professional activities (prebriefing, etc)

supervision, transitions in care, well-being, and health care quality and health care disparities.[26,27] To enact change, the ACGME is providing funding to health care systems and hospitals for participation, again highlighting how important investment at major organizational levels is to creating change. Initiatives such as PEI allows for communication between hospitals and health care systems and will continue to help model processes to change patient safety and culture of safety.

Education on patient safety and on safety culture must be integrated into the curriculum and modeled by health care leaders. Teaching in medical schools and residency should be designed to reflect the importance of safety culture within health care and surgery.[4] If the educational program is grounded in a culture of safety and continuous improvement, physicians are more likely to include these as facets of their own practice after training.[28] Several curricula on quality and safety culture have been developed and include content such as focus on "near miss" events to promote discussions of patient safety and culture of safety, specific teaching on how to properly divulge information regarding medical errors, and leadership training.[29–35] It is important to educate future surgeons holistically, and we gain progress on the longevity of programs and culture change when educational programs incorporate the tools necessary to promote a culture of surgical safety.

Measurement is a key tool to the process of change.[17,36] To properly assess the culture of safety at a given institution, it is important to select a tool that fits. This fit should consider the employee who is receiving the evaluation, and it should provide data on benchmarks as compared with other hospitals and health care systems.[17] Furthermore, proper survey administration and analysis should be used. The Safety Attitudes Questionnaire (SAQ) was adapted from the Flight Management Attitudes Questionnaire and the Cockpit Management Attitudes Questionnaire in aviation.[37–39] The SAQ measures 6 domains, including safety climate and teamwork climate, and provides benchmarks so that institutions can compare themselves with national averages.[37] Identifying variations across health care institutions, and across subspecialties within each individual institution, can help hospitals to learn from errors and to, in turn, ignite change.[40]

Several existing tools designed to improve patient safety may also confer opportunities to establish or improve the culture of safety. The most widely used safety tool in surgery is the surgical checklist. Modeled off of the preflight checklist from the aviation world, the World Health Organization (WHO) Safer Surgery Checklist gives a global standard to safety within operating rooms.[41] This tool, although widely used, does not confer safety without buy-in from stakeholders.[42,43] So, does a culture of safety make employees more likely to use safety checklists? Or, does the requirement to complete safety checklists in turn influence the culture of patient safety? Both are likely true, and investment to create easily-to-follow and institutional-specific checklists can both protect patients and change culture.

The surgical time-out is another commonly used patient safety effort designed to reduce errors. And, as the checklist, another associated benefit of the timeout includes improved safety culture.[44] Some institutions have taken the time out a step further and are including patients in a formal "prebrief or huddle" before surgery.[45] These meetings allow an environment in which any team member can speak up and expectations can be discussed. Following operations, a debrief is a useful tool, even when there is no error or event. When debriefs are commonplace in the surgical environment, conversations are more comfortable. This creates a positive and constructive culture even when there is a safety event to discuss. This focus on regular communication builds team morale and shapes the culture toward one of continued learning and improvement. But, each intervention in isolation is not as powerful as a commitment to using multiple tools to improve patient safety and change culture. The combination of prebriefings, checklists, and debriefings together has been shown to improve safety culture.[46]

Event reporting systems are now used by most hospitals to gather data with regard to patient safety concerns. It is important, though, to recognize that there is the potential for these systems to seem punitive and work against positive culture of safety. Hospitals must work to move away from "blame and shame" cultures and toward a just culture of safety, in which there is support and recognition that errors are inevitable.[17,47] These reporting systems can be valuable tools to help predict and prevent future errors, and improve on current care, as long as they are used within a supportive environment. These reporting systems do not work if employees do not feel a culture of safety and instead abide by a "code of silence."[17] If an individual is blamed when an error is reported, this does little to make change and improve the safety of the system as a whole.[1] Creating a way to report events without retribution is an important facet of any reporting system.[43] If used appropriately, reporting systems create a positive culture of reporting and may provide meaningful information on the real institutional culture and drive forward progress toward a culture of learning and consequent advancement.[47,48]

A culture of safety should be the core of every hospital and health care system. Although enacting change to shift a culture toward one of safety in an established health care system or hospital is an ongoing process, a culture of safety should also be considered when designing new hospitals and systems. If possible, a culture of safety should be at the forefront of the engineering of new health care spaces and hospitals.[49] Social engineering can create a culture of safety encompassing a reporting culture (with a blame-free environment), a learning culture (focused on improving), a just culture (which is fair to all involved), and an informed culture (in which all stakeholders have a general understanding of how their hospital compares between

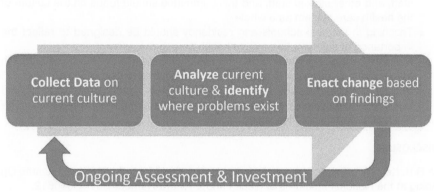

Fig. 1. Advancing surgical safety culture.

national averages and benchmarks).[47] And, by focusing on patient safety as a whole (through interventions such as technology to minimize human error and avoiding reliance on memory when able), safety culture improves as well. Systems improvements decrease stress and make flow easier.[50] Furthermore, patients and patient's families should not only be considered in the engineering but included along with all of the other stakeholders mentioned in the beginning of this article.[49]

SUMMARY

Overall, there is no "silver bullet" solution to create a culture of safety. The process often begins with a measurement of the current culture, strategy development to move behaviors and attitudes to those aligned with a culture of safety, and an investment in the infrastructure necessary to enact positive change (**Fig. 1**). This is a continuous process that must be monitored through recurrent measurement and refinement. Investment at all levels in terms of focus and finance, and ongoing evaluation, are key in creating cultural change and then maintaining it.

In this article, several key processes have been discussed (**Table 1**). Organizations must make safety and a culture of safety part of the mission and core values of a health care system or hospital. Leaders must be established at all levels and must be able to invest resources in changing the culture. Proper communication and education tools must be available, and continuous measurement with proper technique is essential. Checklists, prebriefs, time-outs, debriefs, and event reporting systems, when used appropriately, can both reduce technical errors and change the culture. And finally, when designing new hospitals and health care systems, a culture of safety should be considered a major facet of the engineering and design. As systems invest more focus on a culture of patient safety, we can continue to learn from innovations across the country. There is much promise in future culture, and it is hoped that it will lead to better outcomes for our patients.

CLINICS CARE POINTS

- A culture of surgical safety requires devotion of the leadership to the safety mission, including dedicated time, focus, and financial investment.
- Beyond the organizational leadership, there should be a committee on patient safety and advisory boards, which include supervisors, middle managers, risk managers, safety officers, quality improvement officers, physician staff, nursing

staff, and other clinical staff, and this committee should focus on the culture of the health care system as a whole.
- Teaching in medical schools and residency should be designed to reflect the importance of safety culture within health care and surgery.
- Measurement is a key tool to the process of change, the SAQ is a useful tool in this regard and provides information on benchmarks to help guide change.
- Specific tools, such as checklists, prebriefs, debriefs, executive walk rounds, and event reporting systems can help to create a culture of patient safety, but no individual tool will work in isolation.

DISCLOSURE

Dr R.R. Kelz reports that she receives research support from the National Institute On Aging at the National Institutes of Health under Award Number R01AG060612.

REFERENCES

1. Kohn LT, Corrigan JM, Donaldson MS, et al. To err is human: building a safer health system. Washington, DC: National Academies Press (US); 2000.
2. ASC Communications 2020. 6 elements of a true patient safety culture. In: Becker's Clinical Leadership and Infection Control. 2012. Available at: https://www.beckershospitalreview.com/quality/6-elements-of-a-true-patient-safety-culture.html. Accessed February 15, 2020.
3. The Joint Commission. Improving patient and worker safety: opportunities for synergy, collaboration and innovation. Oakbrook Terrace (IL): The Joint Commission; 2012. Available at: http://www.jointcommission.org/.
4. Fan C, Pawlik T, Daniels T, et al. Association of safety culture with surgical site infection outcomes. J Am Coll Surg 2016;222:122–8.
5. Berry JC, Davis JT, Bartman T, et al. Improved safety culture and teamwork climate are associated with decreases in patient harm and hospital mortality across a hospital system. J Patient Saf 2020;16(2):130–6.
6. Mardon RE, Khanna K, Sorra J, et al. Exploring relationships between hospital patient safety culture and adverse events. J Patient Saf 2010;6(4):226–32.
7. Weaver SJ, Lubomski LH, Wilson RF, et al. Promoting a culture of safety as a patient safety strategy: a systematic review. Ann Intern Med 2013;158(5 Pt 2): 368–74.
8. Sacks GD, Shannon EM, Dawes AJ, et al. Teamwork, communication and safety climate: a systematic review of interventions to improve surgical culture. BMJ Qual Saf 2015;24(7):458–67.
9. The Joint Commission. Safety culture assessment: improving the survey process. The Joint Commission Perspectives. 2018; 38(6).
10. Institute of Medicine (US) Committee on Quality of Health Care in America. In: Kohn LT, Corrigan JM, Donaldson MS, editors. To err is human: building a safer health system. Washington, DC: National Academies Press (US); 2000. https://doi.org/10.17226/9728. Available at: https://www.ncbi.nlm.nih.gov/books/NBK225182/.
11. Russell TR, Jones RS. American college of surgeons remains committed to patient safety. Am Surg 2006;72(11):1005–9.
12. Crutchfield N, Roughton JE. Safety culture: an innovative leadership approach. Oxford: Butterworth-Heinemann; 2013.
13. Hellings J, Schrooten W, Klazinga NS, et al. Improving patient safety culture. Int J Health Care Qual Assur 2010;22(5):489–506.

14. VHA/American Hospital Association (AHA). Strategies of leadership: an organizational approach to patient safety. Oakbrook Terrace (IL): American Hospital Association; 2001. Item # 166925.
15. Makary M, Sexton J, Freischlag J, et al. Patient Safety in Surgery. Ann Surg 2006; 243:628–35.
16. CANSO. Safety culture definition and enhancement process. In: Civil Air Navigation Services Organisation. 2008. Available at: https://www.canso.org/sites/default/files/Safety%20Culture%20Definition%20and%20Enhancement%20Process.pdf. Accessed February 15, 2020.
17. Nieva V, Sorra J. Safety culture assessment: a tool for improving patient safety in healthcare organizations. Qual Saf Health Care 2003;ii:17–22.
18. Sexton J, Sharek P, Thomas E, et al. Exposure to leadership walk rounds in neonatal intensive care units is associated with a better patient safety culture and less caregiver burnout. BMJ Qual Saf 2014;23:814–22.
19. Frankel A, Graydon-Baker E, Neppl C, et al. Patient safety leadership Walk-Rounds. Jt Comm J Qual Saf 2003;29(1):16–26.
20. Auer C, Schwendimann R, Koch R, et al. How hospital leaders contribute to patient safety through the development of trust. J Nurs Adm 2014;44(1):23–9.
21. Keats JP. Leadership and teamwork: essential roles in patient safety. Obstet Gynecol Clin North Am 2019;46(2):293–303.
22. Cooper M, Makary M. A comprehensive unit-based safety program (CUSP) in surgery: improving quality through transparency. Surg Clin North Am 2012;92: 51–63.
23. Makary M, Sexton J, Freischlag J, et al. Operating room teamwork among physicians and nurses: teamwork in the eye of the beholder. J Am Coll Surg 2006;202: 746–52.
24. Thomas L, Galla C. Building a culture of safety through team training and engagement. BMJ Qual Saf 2013;22(5):425–34.
25. Weiss KB, Bagian JP, Nasca TJ. The clinical learning environment: the foundation of graduate medical education. JAMA 2013;309(16):1687–8.
26. Weiss KB, Bagian JP, Wagner R, et al. Introducing the CLER pathways to excellence: a new way of viewing clinical learning environments. J Grad Med Educ 2014;6(3):608–9.
27. Wagner R, Weiss KB, Passiment ML, et al. Pursuing excellence in clinical learning environments. J Grad Med Educ 2016;8(1):124–7.
28. Chen C, Petterson S, Phillips R, et al. Spending patterns in region of residency training and subsequent expenditures for care provided by practicing physicians for Medicare beneficiaries. JAMA 2014;312(22):2385–93.
29. Sachdeva AK, Blair PG. Educating surgery residents in patient safety. Surg Clin North Am 2004;84(6):1669–98.
30. Spencer FC. Human error in hospitals and industrial accidents: current concepts. J Am Coll Surg 2000;191(4):410–8.
31. Crook ED, Stellini M, Levine D, et al. Medical errors and the trainee: ethical concerns. Am J Med Sci 2004;327(1):33–7.
32. ACS NSQIP. Practical QI: the basics of quality improvement. In: The Quality in Training Initiative: an ACS NSQIP Collaborative. 2017. Available at: https://qiti.acsnsqip.org/ACS_NSQIP_2017_QITI_Curriculum.pdf. Accessed May 1, 2020.
33. Sellers MM, Fordham M, Miller CW, et al. The quality in-training initiative: giving residents data to learn clinical effectiveness. J Surg Educ 2018;75(2):397–402.

34. Sellers MM, Reinke CE, Kreider S, et al. American College of Surgeons national surgical quality improvement program's quality in training initiative pilot study. J Surg Res 2013;179(2):231.
35. Kelz RR, Sellers MM, Merkow R, et al. Defining the content for a quality and safety in surgery curriculum using a nominal group technique. J Surg Educ 2019;76(3): 795–801.
36. Campione J, Famolaro T. Promising practices for improving hospital patient safety culture. Jt Comm J Qual Patient Saf 2018;44(1):23–32.
37. Sexton JB, Helreich RL, Neilands TB, et al. The Safety Attitudes Questionnaire: psychometric properties, benchmarking data, and emerging research. BMC Health Serv Res 2006;6(1):44.
38. FMAQ, Helmreich RL, MErrit AC, Sherman JP, et al. The Flight management attitudes Questionnaire (FMAQ). Austin (TX): University of Texas NASA/UT/FAA; 1993. p. 93–4.
39. CMAQ, Helmreich RL. Cockpit management attitudes. Hum Factors 1984;26: 583–9.
40. Pimentel M, Choi S, Fiumara K, et al. Safety culture in the operating room: variability among perioperative healthcare workers. J Patient Saf 2017. https://doi.org/10.1097/PTS.0000000000000385.
41. WHO. Surgical Safety Checklist. In: Patient Safety A World Alliance of Safer Health Care. 2009. Available at: https://www.who.int/patientsafety/safesurgery/checklist/en/. Accessed February 15, 2020.
42. Borchard A, Swappach DLB, Barbir A, et al. A systematic review of the effectiveness, compliance, and critical factors for implementation of safety checklists in surgery. Ann Surg 2012;256:925–33.
43. Mascherek AC, Schwappach DLB, Bezzola P. Frequency of use and knowledge of the WHO-surgical checklist in Swiss hospitals: a cross-sectional online survey. Patient Saf Surg 2013;7(1):36.
44. DeFontes J, Subida S. Preoperative safety briefing project. Perm J 2004;8:21–7.
45. Makary M, Holzmueller C, Thompson D, et al. Operating room briefings: working on the same page. Jt Comm J Wual Paitent Saf 2006;32:351–5.
46. Hill M, Roberts M, Alderson M, et al. Safety culture and the 5 steps to safer surgery: an intervention study. Br J Anesth 2015;114(6):958–62.
47. Reason J. Managing the risks of organizational accidents. London (UK): Ashgate Publishing Limited; 1997.
48. Sellers MM, Berger I, Myers JS, et al. Using patient safety reporting systems to understand the clinical learning environment: A content analysis. J Surg Educ 2018;75(6):e168–77.
49. Reiling J. Creating a culture of patient safety through innovative hospital design. Adv Patient Saf 2005;2:425–39.
50. ASC Communications 2020. How hospitals can improve the culture of safety in the surgical suite: 10 interventions to mitigate risk and create a culture of safety in the OR. In: Becker's Clinical Leadership and Infection Control. 2013. Available at: https://www.beckershospitalreview.com/quality/how-hospitals-can-improve-the-culture-of-safety-in-the-surgical-suite-10-interventions-to-mitigate-risk-and-create-a-culture-of-safety-in-the-or.html. Accessed February 15, 2020.

Effective Implementation and Utilization of Checklists in Surgical Patient Safety

Nikhil Panda, MD, MPH[a,b], Alex B. Haynes, MD, MPH[b,c],*

KEYWORDS

• Surgical safety checklists • Patient safety • Implementation science

KEY POINTS

• The introduction of checklists to enhance the performance of surgical teams has been associated with significant decreases in postoperative mortality and adverse events.
• The differential effect of checklists on patient outcomes in various settings may be due, in part, to strategies for implementation.
• A review of large-scale efforts to introduce checklists in different health systems around the world provides an opportunity to assess the best practices for effective implementation.

INTRODUCTION

The quality of surgical care delivery continues to improve worldwide. Demands for evidence-based and patient-centered surgical care have been met with process improvement, scientific and technological advancements, and even entire restructuring of health systems. Each innovation, however, may add increased complexity to day-to-day workflows, provide challenges to clinicians as they navigate patient care, and ultimately threaten patient safety. Errors continue to occur, each with a significant impact on patient outcomes and quality of life. The introduction of tools to support teams within complex systems first emerged outside of the health care industry and were found to lower preventable errors and minimize harm.

In the last 2 decades, surgeons began adopting checklists as a tool to enhance the performance of surgical teams, minimize adverse events, and improve the survival of patients undergoing surgery. In 2008, the World Health Organization Safe Surgery

[a] Department of Surgery, Massachusetts General Hospital, 55 Fruit Street, Boston, MA 02114, USA; [b] Ariadne Labs, Brigham and Women's Hospital, Harvard T.H. Chan School of Public Health, 401 Park Drive, 3rd Floor West, Boston, MA 02215, USA; [c] Department of Surgery and Perioperative Care, Dell Medical School, The University of Texas at Austin, 1601 Trinity Street, Building B, Austin, TX 78712, USA
* Corresponding author. Department of Surgery and Perioperative Care, Dell Medical School, The University of Texas at Austin, 1601 Trinity Street, Building B, Austin, TX 78712.
E-mail address: Alex.Haynes@austin.utexas.edu
Twitter: @NikhilPanda_MD (N.P.); @masstransitalex (A.B.H.)

Surg Clin N Am 101 (2021) 37–48
https://doi.org/10.1016/j.suc.2020.08.010
0039-6109/21/© 2020 Elsevier Inc. All rights reserved.

Saves Lives initiative introduced a 19-item checklist and piloted it in 8 hospitals around the world, demonstrating a significant decrease in surgical mortality and postoperative complications (**Fig. 1**).[1] In the decade since, versions of surgical checklists have been adapted and introduced into various clinical settings across diverse health systems around the world. Although many initiatives began as similar pilot studies testing the effect of checklists on process measures and patient outcomes, today, checklists have become a part of routine surgical care. In the most recent pooled analysis, it was estimated that 75% of the operating rooms in 94 countries use a surgical checklist in elective care.[2]

Why and how checklists are associated with improvement in clinical outcomes goes back to their original intent: to support the performance of surgical teams by promoting practices that prioritize patient safety. In many settings, incorporating a surgical checklist has been associated with improved perceptions of safety, teamwork, interpersonal communication, and operating room efficiency.[3] In brief, the adoption of checklists has demonstrated that over time aspects of surgical culture can change. But not every experience introducing checklists into surgical practice at scale has resulted in notable improvements in clinical outcomes or team performance. Differences in outcomes may ultimately reflect the underlying implementation strategy. When the introduction of checklists is accomplished through a structured and collaborative approach with engagement from end-users at every level of the health system, checklists seem to be associated with better patient outcomes.

To illustrate this phenomenon, we present and discuss 5 cases describing the large-scale implementation of checklists in different health systems around the world. There are many examples within and outside the practice of surgery that illustrate effective

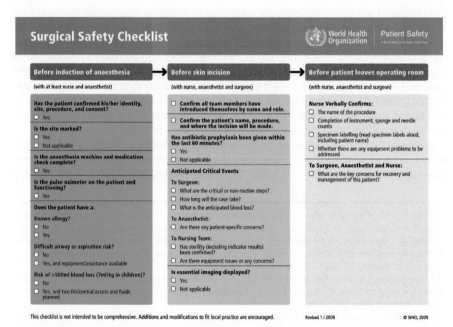

Fig. 1. The World Health Organization surgical safety checklist (2009). (*Courtsey of* World Health Organization, Geneva, Switzerland. Available at: https://www.who.int/patientsafety/safesurgery/checklist/en/.)

implementation of checklists into clinical practice; as such, the included cases are not meant to be exhaustive or comprehensive. The purpose of each case is to highlight strategies, rooted in principles of implementation science, and how each may be associated with differential effects of checklist use on patient outcomes.

CASE PRESENTATIONS
Case 1: The Veteran Health Administration Medical Team Training Program
Background
In 2006, the Veteran Health Administration (VHA) formally launched a previously piloted Medical Team Training Program nationwide.[4] The program was designed to improve patient safety by incorporating checklists that promoted preoperative briefing and postoperative debriefing among operating room staff. At the time of the program launch, the VHA hospitals included 130 facilities offering surgery to millions of patients enrolled within the health system.

Implementation strategy
Initially, the Medical Team Training Program was offered to all VHA health systems in 2006 for voluntary participation. However, after piloting the intervention, the VHA leadership subsequently required facilities to participate in early 2007. Programs were scheduled to participate based on readiness to implement the components of the Medical Team Training Program, rather than using facility-level outcomes data (eg, VHA Surgical Quality Improvement Program data).

The VHA Medical Team Training Program included 3 structured components. The first component was a 2-month period where the program's leadership worked closely with site-specific implementation teams to introduce the program and structure the subsequent phases of implementation. Resources including example checklists, as well as briefing and debriefing tools, were made available to participating facilities. This allowed each facility to actively participate in the implementation process by designing interventions informed by the facility's needs, capabilities, and organizational culture.

The second component was an in-person, day-long introduction of the program and training session. Participants included members of the operating room team, including the surgeons, nurses, anesthesiologists, nurse anesthetists, and operating room technicians. To maximize attendance, no elective cases were scheduled on the date of training. The training session included didactics; simulations including checklist use, briefings, and debriefings; and videos.

The third component of implementation was a series of quarterly telephone-based semistructured interviews with each facility for 1 year after the initial in-person training session. The contact at the facility was a member of the operating room team or member of the hospital administrative leadership (eg, chief of surgery and nursing manager). The purposes of these interviews were to provide support and further guidance for implementation of the Medical Team Training Program, and also to assess effectiveness of the implementation.

Outcomes
In 2010, Neily and colleagues[4] published the results of the VHA Medical Team Training Program in terms of surgical outcomes using VHA Surgical Quality Improvement Program data from 2006 to 2008. Among 108 facilities, 74 participated in the training program and observed an 18% decrease in 30-day surgical mortality compared with baseline patient outcomes. The 34 programs that did not participate observed a decrease in 30-day surgical mortality of 7% compared with baseline. The authors

found that participation in each additional quarter of implementation follow-up (ie, telephone-based semistructured interviews) was associated with a reduction in surgical mortality rates by 0.5 per 1000 deaths. Likewise, higher self-reported quality briefing and debriefing were associated with a reduction in surgical mortality rates by 0.6 per 1000 deaths. Facilities that participated in the Medical Team Training program reported perceptions of better communication, increased awareness, and improved teamwork.

Summary
The structured and coordinated implementation of a checklist-based team training program across VHA facilities was associated with improvements in surgical mortality and perceptions of enhanced teamwork among members of the operating team.

Case 2: The Checklist Mandate in Ontario, Canada

Background
Following the results of the World Health Organization's global pilot study introducing its surgical safety checklist in 8 hospitals, there was enthusiasm for implementing the use of checklists in health systems at scale.[5] In Ontario, Canada, hospitals began rapidly implementing surgical checklists in response to a mandate from the Ontario Ministry of Health and Long-Term Care, stating that all hospitals in the province must begin public reporting of checklist use by July 2010.

Implementation strategy
Given the short amount of time between the 2009 publication of encouraging results from the initial World Health Organization trial and the mandated checklist reporting by July 2010, there was no structured implementation process to introduce checklists to the 133 hospitals performing surgery in Ontario. However, the World Health Organization resources were made available to all hospitals, as were modified versions of the original 19-item checklist, such the Canadian Patient Safety Institute Checklist. Hospitals were encouraged to develop local educational or training sessions as they introduced checklists at their facilities.

The quality of the checklist use was determined through self-report from an individual in the operating room for each procedure. This person was most often a member of the clinical care team, such as a circulating nurse. Compliance across individual procedures was compiled at the hospital level and reported back to the Ministry of Health and Long-Term Care.

Outcomes
The early clinical outcomes from the introduction of the surgical safety checklist in Ontario were published in *The New England Journal of Medicine* in 2014, 5 years after the original 2009 report.[5] Urbach and colleagues present a pre/post analysis during a period of 3 months before and after the rapid implementation of checklists. Among 101 participating surgical hospitals, 79 used the Canadian Patient Safety Institute Checklist. Nine used a customized checklist and four used the original World Health Organization checklist. Ninety-six percent of hospitals included in data analysis reported using an education program during the implementation of their checklists.

Regarding clinical outcomes, the authors reported no difference in risk-adjusted 30-day surgical mortality before (0.71%) and after (0.65%) implementation of checklists. Similarly, there were no differences in the adjusted risk of surgical complications.

Summary
Following a mandate issued to all surgical hospitals in Ontario, the rapid introduction of checklists through facility-level implementation strategies was not associated with significant improvements in surgical mortality or postoperative complications.

Case 3: Surgical Safety Checklists in Norwegian Surgical Care

Background
During a 10-month period from October 2009 to July 2010, Norway implemented modified versions of the World Health Organization surgical safety checklist into 2 hospital systems using a stepped wedge cluster (ie, by surgical specialty) randomized design.[6,7] This approach to checklist implementation allowed participating Norwegian hospitals to rollout the intervention sequentially over time and, importantly, provide a control group to compare the effect checklists on patient safety outcomes.

Implementation strategy
The implementation of a surgical safety checklist in Norwegian health systems began with adapting the original World Health Organization checklist. The 3 scheduled procedure checks and conversation prompts in the original checklist (eg, before induction of anesthesia, before incision of the skin, and before the patient leaves the operating room) were preserved; however, individual aspects of checklists were adapted to fit the local surgical workflow. In addition, checklists were translated from English into Norwegian.

The organizers of checklist implementation then performed small-scale, pilot testing program, incorporating feedback from operating teams that used checklists just weeks after implementation. Checklists were then rolled out across surgical specialties (eg, general surgery, cardiothoracic surgery, and orthopedic surgery) every 4 weeks through a training program including lectures, videos, translated checklist documents from the World Health Organizations, and direct e-mail communication. After the implementation program, there were individuals in the operating room whose sole responsibility was to assess quality of checklist use. A copy of each checklist also included in the patient chart.

Outcomes
The results from the Norwegian experience implementing the surgical safety checklist in 2 hospitals was published in *The Annals of Surgery* in 2015.[6] Notably, this report represented a significant addition to existing evidence on the effect of checklists in surgical care, as it was the first to use an experimental study design, such as the step wedged cluster randomized controlled trial. Haugen and colleagues[6] report a significant reduction in 30-day complication rates in the 3083 operations where checklists were used compared with the 2212 control operations (11.5% from 19.9%).

Importantly, there was a greater decrease in harm when all parts of checklists were used during the intervention operations, suggesting a dose–response relationship. The authors also reported a decrease in overall observed 30-day surgical mortality rates between the intervention (1.0%) and control groups (1.6%). Although this difference seemed to be clinically meaningful among a study base of more than 5000 operations, the study design was not powered to detect a statistically significant decrease in mortality after operations in which checklists had been implemented.

Summary
In a stepped wedge cluster trial evaluating the introduction of checklists across surgical teams in 2 Norwegian hospitals, the implementation of checklists was associated with a significant decrease in postoperative complications. Through direct

observation of operations that used checklists, greater decreases in harm were observed when all parts of checklists were used.

Case 4: The Scottish Patient Safety Program

Background

The Scottish Patient Safety Program (SPSP) was launched in 2008 as a national quality improvement program.[8] The SPSP aimed to foster a culture of prioritizing patient safety by creating and/or implementing existing evidence-based quality improvement interventions to decrease in-hospital mortality by 15% within 5 years.[9] One of the interventions within perioperative care was implementing of the World Health Organization surgical checklist to improve patient safety before, during, and after surgery.

Implementation strategy

The initiatives within the SPSP, including implementation of the surgical checklist, represented a nationwide mandate. The program partnered with regional and local leaders, such as local health boards, and provided support in the form of resources and strategies for effective implementation. Regional and local leaders were encouraged to engage front-line health care workers, especially those in operating room teams, to prioritize patient safety in every aspect of their work. To do this, leaders often made safety walkarounds through all care areas of the hospital (eg, operating theater, inpatient ward, and pharmacy) to discuss patient safety issues as seen through the eyes of the hospital staff.

The implementation process was coordinated by the national program, but tailored and adapted to local considerations and culture by local implementation teams. Checklists were pilot tested among small groups, which led to modifications that would improve the subsequent larger scale rollout. To prepare operating theater members, the local implementation teams provided educational materials designed for each discipline (eg, surgeons, nurses, and anesthesiologists).

Checklist implementation occurred over a 3-year period from 2008 to 2010. During this time, the SPSP organized nationwide meetings, twice each year, to allow individuals within the perioperative arm to share lessons learned during implementation. In addition, there were monthly check-in calls to assess implementation progress, as well as a monthly progress reports required from each local implementation team. In terms of outcome measurement, the SPSP provided and/or trained care providers in the fundamentals of quality improvement, simplified outcome measurement by standardizing definitions of adverse events, and provided program managers to manage data. These data, in addition to site visits, served as metrics of quality assurance and were used to determine if progress toward the overall mission of the SPSP was being made.

Outcomes

The clinical results from the implementation of the surgical safety checklist in Scotland were published recently in *BJS* in 2019.[8] The authors observed that, before the implementation of checklists (2000–2007), there was an absolute decrease in the mortality rate of 0.003% among patients admitted for a surgical procedure. During (2008–2010) and after implementation (2011–2014), the absolute decrease in the mortality rate was 0.069% and 0.019%, respectively. Overall, from 2000 to 2014 the relative decrease in mortality was 36.6%. The study used a nonsurgical cohort of similar size and demographics as a comparator, in which there were no significant improvements in absolute or relative mortality rates during the same study period.

Summary

As a part of a nationwide mandate, implementation of checklists into surgical care over a 3-year period was executed by local implementation teams and supported by the SPSP. A review of surgical outcomes before and after implementation demonstrated a relative decrease in mortality compared with a nonsurgical cohort.

Case 5: The Safe Surgery South Carolina Program

Background

In 2010, the South Carolina Hospital Association partnered with Ariadne Labs, a joint health system innovation center at Brigham and Women's Hospital and Harvard T.H. Chan School of Public Health, to launch a population-level checklist-based quality improvement program to improve surgical safety.[10] The goal was to improve surgical outcomes by encouraging the use of the World Health Organization surgical safety checklist in every operating room across the state.

Implementation strategy

The Safe Surgery South Carolina program implementation process was designed based on results from prior population-level quality improvement initiatives, as well as the 2008 Institute for Health Improvement Sprint Challenge, a small-scale pilot of checklist implementation and use.[11] The program was designed to be completely voluntary. There were 3 levels of implementation teams formed to support the program: (1) the South Carolina Hospital Association and Ariadne Labs; (2) state-level multidisciplinary leadership teams (eg, clinicians, local leaders, and insurance carrier representatives); and (3) hospital-level teams with representation from each surgical discipline (eg, surgeons, nurses, anesthesiologists, nurse anesthetists, and surgical technicians).

The formation of these teams allowed for a needs and context assessment of each participating hospital. This included assessing baseline perceptions of surgical safety and organizational culture, as well as evaluating if each hospital had the necessary resources to carry out the remainder of the implementation program. Hospital-level implementation teams participated in webinars, teleconferences, and coaching visits to prepare for implementation. A formal decision point to move forward with implementation of checklists was incorporated into the needs assessment for each hospital.

The original World Health Organization checklist was adapted to the local workflows of each hospital. After small-scale pilot testing and revisions, checklist training was introduced for each member of the operating room team. This process occurred initially through remote educational materials, such as webinars, teleconferences, and printed materials. Over time, additional in-person activities were added, including one-on-one education and teamwork training. Hospital-level implementation teams and end-users promoted checklists throughout the perioperative phases of care.

The implementation process included several aspects of quality assurance for checklist use. Direct observers assessed checklist use in the operating theater. The South Carolina Hospital Association and Ariadne Labs coordinated site visits and teleconferences to provide coaching on the quality of implementation and assess progress. Hospital-level leadership teams were provided newsletters and reports outlining their institution's performance. A state-wide conference, held twice each year, was organized to allow state- and hospital-level implementation teams to share successes and barriers identified during the implementation process at their respective facilities. In 2015, a self-certification program was created to allow hospitals who participated in the entire implementation process to publicly report that checklists were used to improve patient safety in every operation within the hospital.

Outcomes

The outcomes from the Safe Surgery South Carolina program were published in the *Annals of Surgery* in 2017 by members of the South Carolina Hospital Association and Ariadne Labs.[10] The authors reported the mortality trends before (2008–2010) and after (2010–2013) completing the structured implementation program. Among 14 hospitals that completed the program, the difference in the risk-adjusted 30-day postoperative mortality rates from 2010 to 2013 was 0.54%, compared with a 0.21% increase among noncompleters during the same time period. This outcome corresponded with a relative decrease in risk-adjusted 30-day postoperative mortality rates of 22%. There was also a greater perception of teamwork and a culture of safety among surgical teams within completer hospitals. These hospitals were also more likely to have participated in webinars and the preoperative culture of safety assessment, identified a local clinical champion for the implementation efforts, and attended an in-person team training event.

The Safe Surgery South Carolina program also studied the ongoing effectiveness of checklists as additional facilities completed the implementation program.[11] Hospitals that completed the program had a greater degree of participation in higher touch implementation activities (eg, coaching visits, teamwork skills training, and in-person meetings) versus others (eg, webinars). The same facilities had a greater degree of participation by leadership (eg, hospital chief executive officers) and physicians, although they identified that the discipline most frequently represented was nursing, accounting for 74% of all interactions with the implementation program.

Summary

The Safe Surgery South Carolina program was a voluntary checklist-based quality improvement program that was associated with a decrease in surgical mortality. A review of the program identified facility characteristics and elements of the implementation strategies associated with successful uptake and use.

DISCUSSION

The 5 cases presented here—the VHA Medial Team Training Program, the checklist mandate in Ontario, the implementation in 2 Norwegian hospitals, the SPSP, and the Safe Surgery South Carolina Program—each allow us to make several observations regarding effective implementation of checklists for the purposes of improving patient safety.

Collaboration

First, checklist implementation must be collaborative. Each of the described implementation strategies had a lead sponsor in the form of a governmental agency or parent organization. The most effective sponsors supported teams at the regional or facility levels. In Scotland, the SPSP partnered with leaders of local health boards and supported local implementation teams for each facility. The VHA Medical Team Training Program implementation process began with months of planning to identify champions within each hospital to tailor and guide the subsequent implementation efforts. In brief, truly collaborative strategies were coordinated and supported by the sponsors, but ultimately executed by the local teams. Structuring implementation in this way also allows sponsoring organizations to gather feedback from each facility, and develop best practices informed by the collective implementation experiences of participating health systems. The introduction of checklists in Ontario and the null findings in terms of effects on patient outcomes raises an important consideration: can externally mandated patient safety or quality improvement initiatives succeed?

Or do these programs only thrive among a select group of facilities? In both the VHA health system and Scotland, the introduction of checklists was also mandated, but was facilitated through a structured implementation process informed by members of the local surgical facilities. This level of collaboration is critical to effective implementation of quality improvement initiatives, as unsupported mandates are associated with poor results, in part owing to indifference and perceived burden among end-users.[12–14]

Readiness for Local Implementation

Second, readiness for local implementation must be assessed. As stated, the original intent of checklist-based quality improvement initiatives is to enhance the performance of surgical teams through changes in day-to-day practice. Therefore, checklists are less like one-off tools in a larger quality improvement toolbox, but rather an instrument to help change culture. To introduce or promote an existing culture of patient safety within a health system, it is critical to assess the baseline organizational culture of each health system.[15] Who are the key stakeholders? What are the capabilities in terms of implementation? What is the level of motivation among the end-users?[16] Are there competing initiatives being implemented concurrently? In the VHA Team Training Program, each facility was allowed to schedule when to introduce the program based on their perceived readiness for implementation. The Safe Surgery South Carolina Program formally surveyed members of each facility to assess organizational culture and perceptions of safety. It can be tempting to require immediate, widespread adoption of quality improvement programs, especially tools like a paper-based checklist that, on first review, seem to be relatively simple. Or else prioritize implementation using performance data to identify low-performing health systems.

Establish Buy-in

Third, engage and empower end-users at every level to establish buy-in. A common component of each of the presented implementation strategies was involving, to varying degrees, end-users of checklists during different phases of implementation. In the VHA Medical Team Training Program, facilities scheduled protected time for the operating room teams to attend the in-person educational sessions without competing clinical interests (eg, no elective surgeries were scheduled). This factor not only allowed members of the operating room to undergo simulation training in their usual teams,[17,18] but it also signaled that the VHA and facility leadership supported the initiative. In the Safe Surgery South Carolina Project, the chief executive officer of every health system opted in to participate in the voluntary program, and those programs that completed the entire implementation program reported a greater degree of involvement from chief executive officers throughout the process. The SPSP engaged leaders of local health boards to prioritize patient safety among the frontline workers through initiatives like the safety walkarounds. Each of these examples shows how establishing buy-in at each level of the traditional hierarchy within the health systems can lead to effective implementation of quality improvement initiatives. A recent study conducted by our research team suggested how incorporating medical students, trainees, and early career providers may also benefit implementation and improve sustainability of tools like checklists.[19]

The Importance of Flexibility

Fourth, one size does not fit all. In all of the presented implementation strategies, the original 19-item World Health Organization checklist was modified to fit the preferences, contexts, and workflows of local surgical teams. Even in the most rapid roll out, such as the Ontario experience, only 4 of the 101 participating hospitals used an unmodified version of the checklist. In a 2018 study reviewing more than 150 checklists in the decade after the introduction of the original World Health Organization checklist, Solsky and colleagues[20] found that every checklist had been modified, most frequently with additional items to reflect process measures (eg, equipment availability), or local priorities (eg, reviewing prophylactic anticoagulation). The formation of facility-level implementation teams with local champions allowed for efficient small-scale piloting of checklists, as well as rapid-feedback and revisions of checklists before larger implementation. The process described by the Norwegian hospitals included piloting with scheduled opportunities for revisions within 2 weeks of the initial pilot. Not only does this process increase the likelihood of success during large-scale implementation, but it also further engages and empowers end-users within each facility. Last, many strategies incorporated a variety of educational materials for training members of the operating team. As described by Berry and colleagues[11] when reviewing implementation efforts in the Safe Surgery South Carolina Program, both low-touch (eg, webinars and teleconferences) and high-touch (eg, in-person training, high-fidelity simulation, and site visits) techniques should be offered.

Prepare for Success and Long-Term Sustainability

Fifth, prepare for success and sustainability after initial implementation. In addition to forming local implementation teams, there were important strategies included in many of the presented implementation plans that were geared toward quality assurance and sustainability. Above all, the fidelity of checklist use should be assessed. The Norwegian and South Carolina strategies incorporated direct observation of checklist use in operating rooms. The Ontario experience used self-reporting. It is difficult to measure the effectiveness of tools like checklists without knowledge of their actual use. In addition, a common theme in many strategies was scheduled follow-up between local implementation teams and sponsoring organizations after large-scale implementation of checklists. For the VHA Team Training Program and the Safe Surgery South Carolina project, follow-up provided an opportunity for the local implementation teams to provide feedback on improvements in patient safety metrics, as well as facilitators of and barriers to successful implementation. The sponsoring organizations could provide ongoing coaching and additional resources throughout implementation. In many experiences, there were intentional efforts to create a community among implementers of checklists. As an example, the SPSP and Safe Surgery South Carolina projects organized biannual convenings to allow champions of local implementation teams to present their experiences implementing checklists.

SUMMARY

Realizing the full potential of patient safety and quality improvement initiatives such as surgical safety checklists requires structured, collaborative, and sustainable implementation strategies. Experiences from introducing checklists into diverse health systems around the world have informed best practices. The focus now is on applying the lessons learned from the implementation of tools like checklists toward the introduction of future patient safety initiatives that extend beyond the operating theater. From enhancing preoperative patient–provider shared decision making[21,22] to improving patient engagement and reducing harm throughout surgical recovery,[23] tools like checklists will continue to emerge. Effective implementation and thoughtful efforts to sustain these efforts will ensure surgical teams can provide the highest quality care for their patients.

CLINICAL CARE POINTS

- The introduction of checklists to support the performance of surgical teams is associated with significant decreases in patient mortality and improvements in communication and teamwork.
- The degree to which checklists can support surgical teams relies on a structured implementation strategy coordinated by experienced sponsors and executed by local teams.
- Previous experiences implementing checklists through population-level quality improvement programs have demonstrated the critical elements to effective implementation of checklists.

DISCLOSURE

The authors have nothing to disclose.

REFERENCES

1. Haynes AB, Weiser TG, Berry WR, et al. A surgical safety checklist to reduce morbidity and mortality in a global population. N Engl J Med 2009;360(5):491–9.
2. Delisle M, Pradarelli JC, Panda N, et al. Variation in the global uptake of the surgical safety checklist. Br J Surg 2020;107(2):e151–60.
3. Molina G, Jiang W, Edmondson L, et al. Implementation of the surgical safety checklist in South Carolina hospitals is associated with improvement in perceived perioperative safety. J Am Coll Surg 2016;222(5):725–36.e5.
4. Neily J, Mills PD, Young-Xu Y, et al. Association between implementation of a medical team training program and surgical mortality. JAMA 2010;304(15): 1693–700.
5. Urbach DR, Govindarajan A, Saskin R, et al. Introduction of surgical safety checklists in Ontario, Canada. N Engl J Med 2014;370(11):1029–38.
6. Haugen AS, Søfteland E, Almeland SK, et al. Effect of the World Health Organization checklist on patient outcomes: a stepped wedge cluster randomized controlled trial. Ann Surg 2015;261(5):821–8.
7. Haugen AS, Søfteland E, Eide GE, et al. Impact of the World Health Organization's surgical safety checklist on safety culture in the operating theatre: a controlled intervention study. Br J Anaesth 2013;110(5):807–15.
8. Ramsay G, Haynes AB, Lipsitz SR, et al. Reducing surgical mortality in Scotland by use of the WHO surgical safety checklist. Br J Surg 2019;106(8):1005–11.
9. Haraden C, Leitch J. Scotland's successful national approach to improving patient safety in acute care. Health Aff (Millwood) 2011;30(4):755–63.
10. Haynes AB, Edmondson L, Lipsitz SR, et al. Mortality trends after a voluntary checklist-based surgical safety collaborative. Ann Surg 2017;266(6):923–9.
11. Berry WR, Edmondson L, Gibbons LR, et al. Scaling safety: the South Carolina surgical safety checklist experience. Health Aff (Millwood) 2018;37(11):1779–86.
12. Conway PH, Mostashari F, Clancy C. The future of quality measurement for improvement and accountability. JAMA 2013;309(21):2215–6.
13. Bion J, Richardson A, Hibbert P, et al. Matching Michigan: a 2-year stepped interventional programme to minimise central venous catheter blood stream infections in intensive care units in England. BMJ Qual Saf 2013;22(2):110–23.

14. Dixon-Woods M, Leslie M, Tarrant C, et al. Explaining matching Michigan: an ethnographic study of a patient safety program. Implement Sci 2013;8(1):70.
15. Panda N, Haynes AB. Studying organizational culture in surgery. Cham (Switzerland): Springer; 2020. p. 97–102. https://doi.org/10.1007/978-3-030-28357-5_9.
16. Atlas initiative | Ariadne labs. Available at: https://www.ariadnelabs.org/areas-of-work/atlas-initiative/. Accessed May 20, 2020.
17. Delisle M, Ward MAR, Pradarelli JC, et al. Comparing the learning effectiveness of healthcare simulation in the observer versus active role: systematic review and meta-analysis. Simul Healthc 2019;14(5):318–32.
18. Delisle M, Pradarelli JC, Panda N, et al. Methods for scaling simulation-based teamwork training. BMJ Qual Saf 2019;29(2):98–102.
19. Panda N, Koritsanszky L, Delisle M, et al. Global survey of perceptions of the surgical safety checklist among medical students, trainees, and early career providers. World J Surg 2020. https://doi.org/10.1007/s00268-020-05518-x.
20. Solsky I, Berry W, Edmondson L, et al. WHO surgical safety checklist modification: do changes emphasize communication and teamwork? J Surg Res 2018; 246:614–22.
21. Panda N, Solsky I, Haynes AB. Redefining shared decision-making in the digital era. Eur J Surg Oncol 2019. https://doi.org/10.1016/j.ejso.2019.07.025.
22. Panda N, Haynes AB. Prioritizing the patient perspective in oncologic surgery. Ann Surg Oncol 2019;6–7. https://doi.org/10.1245/s10434-019-07753-6.
23. Panda N, Solsky I, Huang EJ, et al. Using smartphones to capture novel recovery metrics after cancer surgery. JAMA Surg 2019;1–7. https://doi.org/10.1001/jamasurg.2019.4702.

Standardized Care Pathways as a Means to Improve Patient Safety

Elizabeth Lancaster, MD, Elizabeth Wick, MD*

KEYWORDS

- Safety • Quality • Standardization • Enhanced recovery • Checklist

KEY POINTS

- The electronic health record is a valuable tool for standardization and patient safety; however, it can provide variable results early in the implementation process.
- When partnered with changes in culture, checklists and enhanced recovery programs increase standardization and reduce surgical morbidity and mortality.
- Culture, patient complexity, and rotating trainees can represent challenges to standardization, but need to be prohibitive with thoughtful strategies.

INTRODUCTION

Although standardization is a common tool used in any field requiring consistent, high-quality outcomes, it has not been a term widely used in surgery, or medicine overall, until 2000 when the Institute of Medicine (IOM) published "To Err is Human: Building a Safer Healthcare System."[1] In this publication, the lack of standardization in health care was highlighted; "standardization and simplification are two fundamental human factors principles that are widely used in safe industries and widely ignored in health care."

The justifications for the lack of standardization are many: every specialty is different, each patient is unique, providers are highly trained, to name a few. The bottom line, however, is that this exposure of errors in health care brought new light to the fact that standardization is a critical component of providing effective and safe patient care. Of note, the accelerated transition to the electronic health record (EHR) across the continuum of care has, in many cases, forced standardization of care, even on the unwilling clinician. The Affordable Care Act or "Obama Care" included significant financial incentives for hospitals to adopt EHR (Meaningful Use).[2] Around the same time, checklists, although always used, were highlighted as effective tools to improve communication and teamwork, standardizing care along the way. In addition,

Department of Surgery, University of California, 513 Parnassus Avenue, S-321, San Francisco, CA 94143, USA
* Corresponding author.
E-mail address: Elizabeth.wick@ucsf.edu

Surg Clin N Am 101 (2021) 49–56
https://doi.org/10.1016/j.suc.2020.08.011
0039-6109/21/© 2020 Elsevier Inc. All rights reserved.
surgical.theclinics.com

specialty-specific programmatic efforts within surgery have also hastened the transition. Examples of these include enhanced recovery programs (ERP) best characterized for colorectal surgery and verification programs, the most noted being the longstanding Trauma Verification Program, administered by the American College of Surgeons.

DISCUSSION
Role of the Electronic Health Record in Standardized Care

Since the American Recovery and Reinvestment Act of 2009 was signed into law, EHR have become a necessity and staple of medical practice.[2] EHR have created many unique opportunities for improving patient safety through standardization.

One important change with comprehensive EHR was the standardization of the location of patient information. Before integrated EHR use, information was located in several different locations, some electronic, others not, making it challenging for providers to have consistent and accurate patient information.[3] In addition, EHR allow for efficient monitoring of patient safety issues and events. For example, a group of pediatric surgeons developed an automated interface through which surgeons could identify compliance with 10 surgical site infection processes so issues could be addressed in real time.[4] Within 9 months of implementation, compliance increased from 46% to 72% with a decrease in surgical site infections.

Another unique area where the EHR can improve standardization is with the patient hand-off process. Handoffs can be especially challenging in surgical training programs where they occur frequently and recipients have varying levels of patient care experience. A standardized, electronic hand-off tool, using a previously validated template (I-PASS: illness severity, patient summary, action list, situational awareness and contingency planning, and synthesis) showed a reduction in errors in communication by 50% with improved efficiency when used for high-complexity surgical oncology patients.[5]

Despite the benefits of the EHR in standardizing care for surgical patients, it also presents challenges. One such challenge is the initial learning curve after implementation. A study at a tertiary care teaching hospital measured Surgical Care Improvement Project measures before and after implementation, finding an initial decrease in compliance with subsequent improvement after 3 months.[6] In addition, as health information technology becomes more advanced, it can be challenging to find the resources and expertise to translate clinical practices and quality metrics into the EHR.

Checklists

In 2009, surgeon-author Atul Gawande[7] published *The Checklist Manifesto: Getting it Right*, highlighting the value of checklists in medical care. This publication again brought to the public eye gaps in patient safety and proposed checklists as part of the solution. Before Gawande's book, other groups had implemented checklists to improve patient safety with great success. In 2006, the results of a multi-institutional effort to reduce catheter-related bloodstream infections were published, with a key component of their intervention being a checklist with evidence-based procedures to minimize the risk of contamination and infection.[8] Within the 103 intensive care units studied, this group found a reduction in catheter-related bloodstream infections from 2.7 per 1000 catheter-days to 0 after a 3-month implementation period.

In 2004, the Joint Commission established the Universal Protocol for Preventing Wrong-Site, Wrong-Procedure, and Wrong-Person Surgery, requiring a preprocedure verification process, procedure site marking, and a time-out before starting any invasive procedure.[9] Although not a checklist itself, the protocol requires checklists as part of its implementation; however, to date, studies have not examined its effectiveness in preventing wrong-site, wrong-procedure, or wrong-person surgery.[10]

In 2008, Gawande and colleagues[11,12] developed the Surgical Safety Checklist based on the World Health Organization (WHO) Guidelines for Safe Surgery, implementing and studying its effects in 8 hospitals worldwide. The checklist describes a "sign in" before anesthesia induction, a "time out" before skin incisions, and a "sign out" before the patient leaves the operating room, where specific, critical components of providing safe patient care are identified and addressed. Implementation of this checklist led to a reduction in death from 1.5% to 0.7% and in inpatient complications from 11% to 7%.

With similar goals, the Surgical Patient Safety System (SURPASS) Collaborative Group from the Netherlands studied the implementation of a more comprehensive patient safety surgical checklist at 6 hospitals, comparing changes in patient outcomes to 5 control hospitals.[13] The SURPASS Checklist is transdisciplinary, with items spanning the entire hospital course, including imaging review, equipment/material checks, surgical site marking, postoperative hand-off instructions, and prescriptions provided at discharge. Similar to the WHO Surgical Safety Checklist study, they found a decrease in in-hospital mortality from 1.5% to 0.8% and a decrease in overall complication rate from 27.3 to 16.7 per 100 patients.

Importantly, a checklist, without promotion of teamwork and communication and a culture of safety, will not be effective. Pronovost and colleagues[8] demonstrated the effectiveness of a checklist to reduce central line–associated bloodstream infections, but in the context of a cultural intervention.[14] Hospitals that did not embrace a culture of safety failed to see the same positive impact from checklist adoption as compared with those that did. Based on this work, it has been proposed that improvement in surgery combines both technical interventions (eg, a checklist, pathway, verification program) with adaptive changes (eg, a culture of safety, promotion of speaking up and speaking out, supportive leadership) (**Fig. 1**).

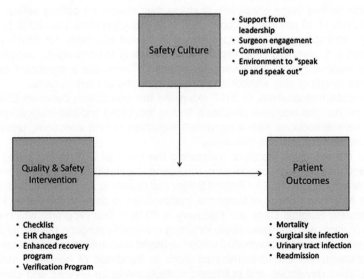

Fig. 1. Safety culture moderates the effectiveness of safety and quality improvement efforts.

Enhanced Recovery Programs

Although not described as "standardized care" per se and not widely disseminated, practices and specialties were engaging in standardization before the IOM publication in 2000. For example, in 1994, Engelman and colleagues[15] described their "fast-track recovery" protocol, a standardized, evidence-based approach to caring for coronary artery bypass graft patients preoperatively, intraoperatively, and postoperatively. This report represents one of the earliest published examples of what would become the wave of ERP, or enhanced recovery after surgery (ERAS). The "Enhanced Recovery" movement, which gained popularity in the 2000s, is centered on providing evidence-based, standardized care to surgical patients in order to improve patient safety and optimize perioperative outcomes.

In 2001, a group from the United Kingdom first coined the term Enhanced Recovery After Surgery, describing key elements of perioperative care for colorectal resections based on best available evidence.[16] The motivation for this consensus review was the wide variation in clinical care following major abdominal surgery, with a particular focus on maintaining "normal" physiology as much as possible throughout the perioperative period: avoiding large shifts in fluids, hyperglycemia and hypoglycemia, and excessive opioids. The proposed pathway was comprehensive: outlining key elements of preoperative, intraoperative, and postoperative care relating to patient counseling, nutrition and fluid balance, management of tubes and drains, infection prophylaxis, and analgesia. This group of academic surgeons went on to form the ERAS Society in 2010, which has published guidelines for colonic resection, rectal resection, pancreaticoduodenectomy, cystectomy, gastric resection, gynecologic surgery, bariatric surgery, head and neck cancer surgery, liver resection, breast reconstruction, hip and knee replacement, thoracic noncardiac surgery, and esophageal resection.[17] Importantly, it was recognized that effective implementation required that ERAS pathways spanned the continuum of care and included buy-in and support from all providers (surgeons, nurses, anesthesia providers) and inherently resulted in standardization. The days of remembering that Dr Jones used ertapenem and Dr Smith used ceftriaxone were inherently over with the proper adoption of ERAS.

Since these first ERAS guidelines, numerous hospitals and groups have adapted and implemented these principles, studying their effects on patient safety. A 2013 metaanalysis of 16 randomized controlled trials including more than 2000 colorectal surgery patients showed an improvement in overall morbidity for ERAS patients compared with standard care, especially with regards to nonsurgical complications, such as respiratory and cardiovascular events.[18] There was a significant decrease in hospital length of stay without an increase in deaths or readmissions.

A separate metaanalysis in 2017 examined the association between ERAS programs and hospital-acquired infections, finding that ERAS and fast-track surgery programs were associated with a significant reduction in lung infections, urinary tract infections, and surgical site infections.[19]

Given the extensive literature supporting the value of ERP in improving patient safety and the quality of surgical care, the Agency for Healthcare Research and Quality, the Armstrong Institute for Patient Safety and Quality at Johns Hopkins University, and the American College of Surgeons, collaborated to develop the Safety Program for Improving Surgical Care and Recovery in 2016.[20] This program, which encompasses multiple surgical specialties, including orthopedic surgery, colorectal surgery, and gynecologic surgery, compiled evidence-based best practices with practical tools for implementation and disseminated them to hundreds of hospitals nationwide (**Fig. 2**). They developed and published multiple evidence reviews and continue to

A Program content requirements

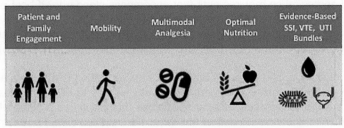

B System requirements

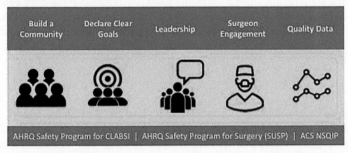

Fig. 2. Program content (*A*) and system (*B*) requirements for successful ERP. SSI, surgical site infections; UTI, urinary tract infections; VTE, venous thromboembolism.

update their program as new data emerge.[21–26] The project is still ongoing, with anticipated completion in 2022. Early examination of data is suggestive that hospital participation is associated with improved patient outcomes, but further data and analysis are needed.

Barriers to Standardization

Although developing ERP and checklists, and integrating them into the EHR may seem like a simple solution to provide standardized, high-quality care, there are many practical barriers to standardization that need to be addressed. A systematic review of 53 articles describing ERP found 3 major barriers to ERP implementation: resistance to change from frontline clinicians, inadequate resources, and external factors, including patient complexity or hospital setting.[27] Resistance to change speaks to the culture of a clinical setting, with studies showing improvements in culture are associated with improvements in clinical outcomes.[28] As discussed previously, improvements in safety attitudes are also essential for improving patient outcomes with checklist implementation.[29] Dedicated effort, however, is necessary to develop a culture that is supportive of evidence-based standardization. For example, implementing an organizational accountability model, with clear expectations from all stakeholders, including hospital leadership, frontline staff, and patients, with regards to responsibility, capacity, and resources, has been shown to reduce surgical site infections, improve patient experience, and decrease costs.[30]

Patient complexity can represent another barrier to providing standardized care, whereby patient care may be more nuanced and less amenable to a checklist or pathway. Many patients with cancer, for example, require multiple specialties and varying treatment pathways depending on their disease stage and comorbidities. Here, innovative methods are necessary for standardizing care and optimizing outcomes. Several specialty societies, such as the Commission on Cancer, have developed accreditation requirements that encompass standardized best practices, including details such as patient navigation and tumor boards.[31] Studies have shown that when thoughtfully designed and implemented, ERAS pathways can be successful in improving patient outcomes even after complex operations, such as open liver resections.[32]

Another challenge, and potential barrier, to standardization is residents and other trainees at academic institutions, particularly with regards to ERP. Trainees tend to rotate on and off of services/surgical specialties multiple times a year, which can make it difficult to continue to deliver the same standardized care. For example, in a study evaluating the effectiveness of dedicated operating teams in an ERAS pathway for colorectal surgery, anesthesia residents were not included in the core ERAS anesthesia team because they were thought to increase variability.[19] Standardized order sets in the EHR, as well as dedicated patient safety and enhanced recovery education, can help incorporate trainees into standardized care pathways rather than exclude them from it.[33]

SUMMARY

The literature overwhelmingly supports standardized, evidence-based care to improve patient safety in the surgical setting, including checklists and ERP. Although local culture, patient complexity, and hospital setting can represent barriers to implanting standardized practices, they can be overcome with thoughtful strategies.

CLINICS CARE POINTS

- The electronic health record is a valuable tool for standardization and patient safety, but careful attention to development and implementation of order sets and pathways is required.
- When partnered with changes in culture, checklists and enhanced recovery programs increase standardization and reduce surgical morbidity and mortality.
- Culture, patient complexity, and rotating trainees can represent challenges to standardization, but can be mitigated with thoughtful strategies.

DISCLOSURE

The authors have nothing to disclose.

REFERENCES

1. Kohn LT, Corrigan J, Donaldson MS. To err is human: building a safer health system. Washington, DC.: National Academy Press; 2000.
2. Burke T. The health information technology provisions in the American Recovery and Reinvestment Act of 2009: implications for public health policy and practice. Public Health Rep 2010;125(1):141–5.
3. Sittig DF, Singh H. Electronic health records and national patient-safety goals. N Engl J Med 2012;367(19):1854–60.
4. Fisher JC, Godfried DH, Lighter-Fisher J, et al. A novel approach to leveraging electronic health record data to enhance pediatric surgical quality improvement bundle process compliance. J Pediatr Surg 2016;51(6):1030–3.
5. Clarke CE, Patel S, Ives N, et al. Clinical effectiveness and cost-effectiveness of physiotherapy and occupational therapy versus no therapy in mild to moderate

Parkinson's disease: a large pragmatic randomised controlled trial (PD REHAB). Health Technol Assess 2016;20(63):1–96.

6. Thirukumaran CP, Dolan JG, Reagan Webster P, et al. The impact of electronic health record implementation and use on performance of the surgical care improvement project measures. Health Serv Res 2015;50(1):273–89.

7. Gwande A. The checklist manifesto: how to get things right. 1st edition. New York: Metropolitan Books; 2009.

8. Pronovost P, Needham D, Berenholtz S, et al. An intervention to decrease catheter-related bloodstream infections in the ICU. N Engl J Med 2006;355(26): 2725–32.

9. Universal protocol for preventing wrong site, wrong procedure, wrong person surgery: JCAHO; Joint Commission on Accreditation of Healthcare Organizations. 2020. Available at: https://www.jointcommission.org/-/media/tjc/documents/standards/universal-protocol/up_poster1pdf.pdf. Accessed April 24, 2020.

10. Treadwell JR, Lucas S, Tsou AY. Surgical checklists: a systematic review of impacts and implementation. BMJ Qual Saf 2014;23(4):299–318.

11. Haynes AB, Weiser TG, Berry WR, et al. A surgical safety checklist to reduce morbidity and mortality in a global population. N Engl J Med 2009;360(5):491–9.

12. WHO guidelines for safe surgery 2009: safe surgery saves lives. WHO; Geneva (Switzerland): 2009.

13. de Vries EN, Prins HA, Crolla RM, et al. Effect of a comprehensive surgical safety system on patient outcomes. N Engl J Med 2010;363(20):1928–37.

14. Bosk CL, Dixon-Woods M, Goeschel CA, et al. Reality check for checklists. Lancet 2009;374(9688):444–5.

15. Engelman RM, Rousou JA, Flack JE 3rd, et al. Fast-track recovery of the coronary bypass patient. Ann Thorac Surg 1994;58(6):1742–6.

16. Fearon KC, Ljungqvist O, Von Meyenfeldt M, et al. Enhanced recovery after surgery: a consensus review of clinical care for patients undergoing colonic resection. Clin Nutr 2005;24(3):466–77.

17. Ljungqvist O, Scott M, Fearon KC. Enhanced recovery after surgery: a review. JAMA Surg 2017;152(3):292–8.

18. Greco M, Capretti G, Beretta L, et al. Enhanced recovery program in colorectal surgery: a meta-analysis of randomized controlled trials. World J Surg 2014; 38(6):1531–41.

19. Grant MC, Hanna A, Benson A, et al. Dedicated operating room teams and clinical outcomes in an enhanced recovery after surgery pathway for colorectal surgery. J Am Coll Surg 2018;226(3):267–76.

20. AHRQ safety program for improving surgical care and recovery. Agency for Healthcare Research and Quality. Available at: https://www.ahrq.gov/hai/tools/enhanced-recovery/index.html. Accessed April 20, 2020.

21. Ban KA, Gibbons MM, Ko CY, et al. Surgical technical evidence review for colorectal surgery conducted for the AHRQ safety program for improving surgical care and recovery. J Am Coll Surg 2017;225(4):548–557 e3.

22. Soffin EM, Gibbons MM, Ko CY, et al. Evidence review conducted for the agency for healthcare research and quality safety program for improving surgical care and recovery: focus on anesthesiology for total knee arthroplasty. Anesth Analg 2019;128(3):441–53.

23. Soffin EM, Gibbons MM, Wick EC, et al. Evidence review conducted for the agency for healthcare research and quality safety program for improving surgical care and recovery: focus on anesthesiology for hip fracture surgery. Anesth Analg 2019;128(6):1107–17.

24. Hornor MA, Liu JY, Hu QL, et al. Surgical technical evidence review for acute appendectomy conducted for the agency for healthcare research and quality safety program for improving surgical care and recovery. J Am Coll Surg 2018;227(6): 605–617 e2.

25. Grant MC, Gibbons MM, Ko CY, et al. Evidence review conducted for the agency for healthcare research and quality safety program for improving surgical care and recovery: focus on anesthesiology for bariatric surgery. Anesth Analg 2019;129(1):51–60.

26. Grant MC, Gibbons MM, Ko CY, et al. Evidence review conducted for the AHRQ safety program for improving surgical care and recovery: focus on anesthesiology for gynecologic surgery. Reg Anesth Pain Med 2019. https://doi.org/10. 1136/rapm-2018-100071.

27. Stone AB, Yuan CT, Rosen MA, et al. Barriers to and facilitators of implementing enhanced recovery pathways using an implementation framework: a systematic review. JAMA Surg 2018;153(3):270–9.

28. Sacks GD, Shannon EM, Dawes AJ, et al. Teamwork, communication and safety climate: a systematic review of interventions to improve surgical culture. BMJ Qual Saf 2015;24(7):458–67.

29. Haynes AB, Weiser TG, Berry WR, et al. Changes in safety attitude and relationship to decreased postoperative morbidity and mortality following implementation of a checklist-based surgical safety intervention. BMJ Qual Saf 2011;20(1): 102–7.

30. Wick EC, Galante DJ, Hobson DB, et al. Organizational culture changes result in improvement in patient-centered outcomes: implementation of an integrated recovery pathway for surgical patients. J Am Coll Surg 2015;221(3):669–77 [quiz: 785–6].

31. Wick EC, Cinar P. Variation across the continuum of surgical oncology care. JAMA Netw Open 2018;1(6):e183035.

32. Page AJ, Gani F, Crowley KT, et al. Patient outcomes and provider perceptions following implementation of a standardized perioperative care pathway for open liver resection. Br J Surg 2016;103(5):564–71.

33. Stone AB, Leeds IL, Efron J, et al. Enhanced recovery after surgery pathways and resident physicians: barrier or opportunity? Dis Colon Rectum 2016;59(10): 1000–1.

Optimizing Safety for Surgical Patients Undergoing Interhospital Transfer

Angela Ingraham, MD, MS[a], Caroline E. Reinke, MD, MSHP[b],*

KEYWORDS

- Interhospital transfer • Interfacility transfer • Transfer outcomes • Patient safety
- Communication

KEY POINTS

- Interhospital transfers of surgical patients pose unique challenges to ensure optimal care.
- Patients who are transferred between hospitals have worse outcomes than directly admitted patients, which may be impacted by gaps in communication and a lack of coordination of care between referring and accepting providers.
- Previous research and quality improvement efforts that focus on other transitions of care may provide insights as to how to optimize transfers between acute care hospitals.

INTRODUCTION

Transitions of care are common and an integral component of modern health care. These transitions can happen during care within a single facility (eg, operating room to intensive care unit [ICU], ICU to floor) or between two health care facilities (eg, discharges from an acute care hospital to a skilled nursing facility, transfers between acute care hospitals). When patients undergo transitions of care, they are vulnerable to gaps in communication and disruptions of their care that can have adverse consequences. Although prior research has investigated interruptions in care and developed best practices for transitions of care within a single facility[1–3] and at discharge to a lower level of care,[4–6] this article focuses on transitions that span across acute care hospitals.

Although much can be learned from the existing literature focusing on transitions of care, transfers of patients with emergent medical, and in particular surgical, needs

[a] Department of Surgery, University of Wisconsin-Madison, G5/342 CSC, 600 Highland Avenue, Madison, WI 53792, USA; [b] Department of Surgery, Carolinas Medical Center, Atrium Health, 1025 Morehead Medical Drive, Suite 300, Charlotte, NC 28204, USA
* Corresponding author.
E-mail address: Caroline.e.reinke@atriumhealth.org
Twitter: @AngieIngrahamMD (A.I.)

Surg Clin N Am 101 (2021) 57–69
https://doi.org/10.1016/j.suc.2020.09.002
0039-6109/21/© 2020 Elsevier Inc. All rights reserved.

between acute care hospitals pose unique challenges and are frequently complex. The care teams are separated in space and also often separated in time. Providers may be documenting and providing care through different medical record systems that may or may not allow cross-communication. Although interhospital transitions are less common, they are not infrequent,[7,8] leaving room for greater vulnerability but also improvement. This article reviews prior research on the epidemiology and outcomes for surgical patients who undergo interhospital transfer, describes the complexities inherent to this process, and reviews gaps in current knowledge. Needs for future research is outlined and best practices from other transitions of care scenarios are reviewed to identify aspects that could be modified for interhospital transfers.

INTERHOSPITAL TRANSFERS: EPIDEMIOLOGY AND REASONS FOR TRANSFER

In 2009, almost 1.4 million patients underwent interhospital transfer within in the National Inpatient Sample, which represented 4% of the overall National Inpatient Sample population, and increased annually by 1.56% from 1993 to 2009.[9] This reported rate of interhospital transfer is similar in surgical populations and has increased over time. In the emergency general surgery population, interhospital transfer increased from just more than 1% to 3% between 2002 and 2011 (**Fig. 1**).[10] Comparing the rate of interhospital transfers using the American College of Surgeons National Surgery Quality Improvement Program database, transfers of patients who underwent surgery increased from 3.2% between 2005 and 2008 to 4.5% between 2009 and 2012.[11]

Use of Interhospital Transfer in Specific Patient Populations

The application of standardized processes for interhospital transfer is best described in the care of patients suffering trauma, acute myocardial infarction, and stroke.[12-17] Regionalization of trauma care began in the 1970s.[18] Studies in this population in

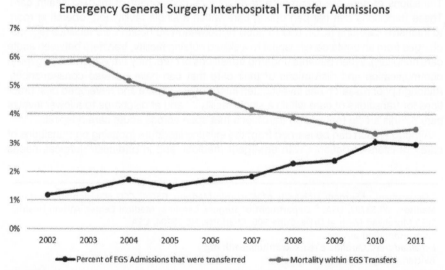

Fig. 1. Trends in emergency general surgery (EGS) interhospital transfers. (*From* Reinke CE, Thomason M, Paton L, et al. Emergency general surgery transfers in the United States: a 10-year analysis. J Surg Res. 2017;219:128-135; with permission.)

the late 1990s and early 2000s suggested improved outcomes for trauma patients managed in trauma centers (relative risk, 0.80; 95% confidence interval [CI], 0.60–0.95) and improved mortality after regionalization (52% preregionalization vs 18% in phase II of regionalization).[12,13] More recently, a meta-analysis of 36 observational studies noted no difference in mortality for patients managed at trauma centers between those that were transferred and those that were directly admitted (relative risk, 1.06; 95% CI, 0.90–1.25).[19] However, the authors of that meta-analysis noted that conclusive judgements regarding the impact of interhospital transfer on mortality after major trauma could not be made because of substantial heterogeneity across studies and that most studies excluded patients dying at outlying hospitals.

Regionalization for acute medical diagnoses, such as myocardial infarction and stroke, has developed in response to data suggesting that time-sensitive procedural intervention (percutaneous catheterization or endovascular treatment) improves patient outcomes. This has resulted in increased rates of interhospital transfer for patients with these diagnoses.[14,20] These patient populations have a specific single medical diagnosis that can be treated with a unique, specific procedural intervention that is recommended as a best practice but not available at all hospitals.

In contrast, surgical transfers involve a broad spectrum of diagnoses and interventions, surgeries, and procedures that are done by interventional colleagues, such as interventional radiology and gastroenterology. Thus, the depth, breadth, and complexity of surgical patients who are transferred varies. Interhospital transfers of surgical patients occur frequently,[10,11] and the diagnoses, reasons for transfer, and outcomes vary.[21] Opportunities to standardize the transfer process exist, and doing so is likely to benefit the patient, surgeons, hospitals, and the US health care system.

As the surgical community has made advances in processes for the triage of trauma patients, medical knowledge around surgical critical care, and other options for nonoperative management (advanced gastroenterology, interventional radiology), it is not surprising that the incidence of interhospital transfers for surgical patients has increased. Yet, despite the increased cost and potential for gaps in care and clinical decline while awaiting or during transfer,[22–24] this process remains highly variable by facilities and by individual providers involved in the process. Coordinated transfers based on creation of standardized guidelines and processes, referred to commonly as regionalization, have been advocated as a method to address shortages of emergency general surgery clinical coverage and increase revenue streams.[25,26]

Reasons for Transfer of Surgical Patients

Although the interhospital transfer process may have initially been more influenced by patient's ability to pay rather than severity of illness,[27] interhospital transfers of surgical patients are most commonly performed now to best match patient needs with hospital resources.[28] The reasons that surgical patients are transferred are numerous and multifactorial. Caring for surgical patients necessitates collaboration between multiple health care team members (nurses, physician extenders, physicians [emergency medicine, anesthesia, surgery, and other specialties]) and a wide array of physical resources (imaging technology, operating room facilities, and procedure rooms).[28] Referring hospitals and providers may not have the necessary resources to care for a patient (**Table 1**).

Additionally, patients and/or their families may request to be transferred to a different facility for a myriad of reasons (eg, favorable or unfavorable experience with either of the hospitals, proximity to loved ones, continuity of care). One qualitative study of transferred patients identified that requests to transfer were influenced by the quality of care; severity and potential consequences of the illness; and the patient's

Table 1	
Potential factors impacting a hospital's ability to care for a patient with a surgical diagnosis	
Category	**Examples (Not All-Inclusive)**
Physical resources	Bed availability Level of care Dialysis units
Diagnostic capabilities	Computerized tomography capability MRI capability
Consulting services	General surgery Surgical subspecialties Infectious disease Nephrology Critical care
Procedural services	Interventional radiology Gastroenterology
Staffing	Patient/nurse ratios Operating room nurses and surgical technicians

relationship with community hospitals, physicians, and tertiary care facilities (**Fig. 2**).[29] Finally, providers at the referring facility may determine that the patient's needs (whether because of preexisting comorbidities or the severity of the acute illness) exceed that which can be cared for at their facility or would be best cared for at a different location.

Factors Associated with Surgical Transfers

Examining adult emergency general surgery patients in the 2008 to 2013 Nationwide Inpatient Sample, 1.8% of encounters resulted in a transfer out to another acute care hospital. Transferred patients were on average 62 year old, white, and most commonly had Medicare insurance (52.9%). Among transferred patients, the most common

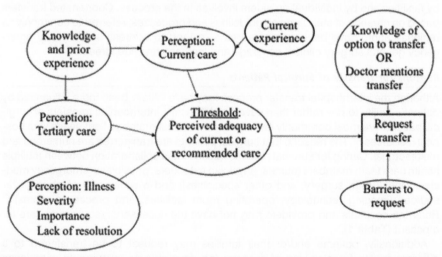

Fig. 2. Influence diagram for patients' and families' perceptions of the decision to transfer to tertiary care. (*From* Dy SM, Rubin HR, Lehmann HP. Why do patients and families request transfers to tertiary care? a qualitative study. Soc Sci Med. 2005;61(8):1846-1853; with permission.)

emergency general surgery diagnoses were related to hepatic-pancreatic-biliary (28.6%) and upper gastrointestinal tract (18.9%) conditions. Most transferred patients (84.8%) did not undergo a procedure before transfer. Transfer was more likely if patients were in small (hazard ratio [HR], 2.52; 95% CI, 2.28–2.79) or medium (HR, 1.32; 95% CI, 1.21–1.44) versus large facilities, government (HR, 1.19; 95% CI, 1.11–1.28) versus private facilities, and rural (HR, 4.58; 95% CI, 3.98–5.27) or urban nonteaching (HR, 1.89; 95% CI, 1.70–2.10) versus urban teaching facilities. These hospital-level characteristics more strongly predicted the need for transfer than patient-related factors.[21] This is in concordance with an earlier single-institution study that concluded that factors beyond patient characteristics, such as lack of surgical access or lack of comfort with more basic surgical patients, are influencing the need for transfer.[30]

INTERHOSPITAL TRANSFERS: ADVERSE OUTCOMES FOR TRANSFERRED PATIENTS

Patients who undergo interhospital transfer have been shown to have increased rates of adverse outcomes in most studies. Increased mortality has been demonstrated in a variety of transferred populations including the broad emergency general surgery[11,31–34] populations, patients with necrotizing fasciitis,[35] and surgical intensive care patients (**Table 2**).[36]

Many of these studies used risk adjustment to attempt to mitigate for the fact that the patients that undergo transfer have greater comorbidities and often greater severity of illness. To our knowledge, no studies exist in which patients are randomized to transfer, and such a study is unlikely to ever be ethical. There are a few studies that demonstrate equivalent outcomes with risk adjustment in the ICU population,[37] for general surgery patients,[38] and for patients with necrotizing fasciitis.[39] It is clear that the population of patients that undergo interhospital transfer are more ill than those that do not. However, it remains unknown what portion of the increased adverse outcomes are caused by patient comorbidities, disease severity, or the actual process of transfer.

Irrespective of patient outcomes, transfers are inherently associated with increased resource use.[30,32,37] For trauma patients, excess care in the form of repeat imaging has been documented, and these findings would likely be similar in other surgical populations.[40,41] In another study of patients transferred from an emergence department to a tertiary care hospital, patients often underwent repeated laboratory tests and radiographic imaging with many (99.5% and 73.6%, respectively) being deemed inappropriate.[42]

INTERHOSPITAL TRANSFERS: INHERENT COMPLEXITIES

Although every patient care transition has its own complexities and associated vulnerabilities, the interhospital transfer has unique complexities that must be considered. An overview is provided of the most common, impactful complexities, but certainly there are more than can be covered in this space.

The transfer process is labor-intensive with multiple involved stakeholders (**Fig. 3**). The team caring for the patient must initiate the transfer with the accepting hospital, often through a transfer center that may or may not be staffed by individuals with direct patient care experience. Connecting the providers at the referring and accepting hospitals can require multiple telephone calls depending on each provider's current availability. Once a connection is made, referring providers may need to talk to multiple care teams at the accepting facility depending on the specific patient needs and the resources and culture at the accepting facility. For example, hospitals may have a

Table 2
Mortality among surgical patients who are transferred

Author (Year)	Population	Transfer Mortality (%)	Nontransfer Mortality (%)	Risk-Adjusted Mortality (95% CI)	Other Comments
Castillo-Angeles et al,[33] 2020	NSQIP patients undergoing EGS procedures 2005–2014	10.8	3.1	1.01 (1.01–1.02)	Propensity score matched analysis
Yelverton et al,[31] 2018	NIS EGS diagnoses 2002–2011	4.2	1.5	2.34 (2.18–2.54)	Logistic regression analysis
Santry et al,[32] 2011	Single-center review of patients admitted to an ACS service 2006–2009	4.9	0.9	Not significant	Logistic regression analysis
Huntington et al,[11] 2016	NSQIP patients transferred from an outside hospital or emergency department 2005–2012	8.9	1.7	Remained significantly different	Mortality compared between matched cohorts of transferred vs nontransferred
Crippen et al,[34] 2014	UHC broad surgical specialties as discharge physician 2010–2012	5.7	1.8	Not performed	Analyzed local institutional data to evaluate use of high-impact resource categories and cost
Holena et al,[35] 2011	NIS with primary diagnosis of necrotizing fasciitis 2000–2006	15.5	8.7	2.04 (1.60–2.59)	Logistic regression controlling for patient and hospital variables
Arthur et al,[36] 2013	Single institution SICU admission database 2009–2011	—	—	1.60 (1.04–2.45)	Logistic regression controlling for age, ICU length of stay, and APACHE II

Abbreviations: ACS, acute care surgery; APACHE, Acute Physiologic Assessment and Chronic Health Evaluation; EGS, emergency general surgery; NIS, Nationwide Inpatient Sample; NSQIP, National Surgical Quality Improvement Program; SICU, surgical intensive care unit; UHC, UnitedHealthcare.
Data from Refs.[11,31–36]

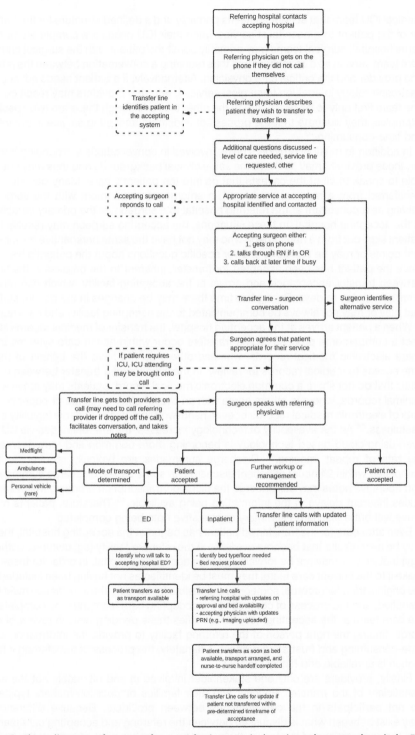

Fig. 3. Flow diagram of process for transferring surgical patients between hospitals. ED, emergency department; OR, operating room.

medical ICU team that accepts patients primarily and a defined structure for the transfer of the patient to a hospitalist service when their ICU needs are completed; at the same hospital, surgical teams may primarily admit the patient with the surgical critical care team serving as a consultant and thus requiring a conversation between the referring provider and the critical care physician. Alternatively, if a patient needs advanced gastroenterology in addition to surgical services, referring providers may reach out to one team first only to be redirected to the other team. Although these are two specific examples, they illustrate that the process of finding an accepting service is complex and time-consuming.[43]

In addition to multiple providers being involved in conversations surrounding transfer, those providers may not have the same clinical backgrounds and thus may not be able to speak to all of the caveats that go into the patient's care. Many patients are transferred from a medical service or an emergency department with the surgeon serving as a consultant at the referring hospital to a surgeon as the primary caregiver at the accepting hospital. In these situations, the accepting surgeon may receive the patient sign-out from a nonsurgeon who may not have the same perspective on important points or may be unable to answer specific questions about the patient's history. Once the patient has been accepted for transfer, inherent to the process is the time between transfer acceptance and arrival at the accepting facility, which can range from 30 minutes to days. During this time there may be changes in the patient status that may or may not always be communicated to the accepting facility and care team.

When a patient arrives at the accepting hospital, the transfer of medical records is at best a cumbersome process. Some transfers occur within health care systems that share electronic medical records, whereas others do not have the benefit of real-time access to medical records for review. In the situation of a transfer between hospitals that do not share a common electronic medical record, patients may arrive with minimal records, whereas others come with an overwhelming volume of paper printouts of electronic medical records or even hand-written notes of variable legibility and usefulness.[44] As the availability of technology increases, transfer of images via CD or even using cloud-based technology is becoming more common and may decrease the rate of repeat imaging.[41] Discharge summaries are typically required to be completed within 24 hours of patient discharge. In some cases, discharge summaries and operative notes may still undergo the dictation/transcription process, which introduces inherent delays in the information being available.[45] Therefore, patients may arrive without a discharge summary or operative note being completed.

Even after care for the transferred patient has begun at the accepting hospital, there may be new results that become available at the referring facility (eg, cultures, pathology) that may or may not be forwarded to the accepting hospital. In order for these to make it to the current care team, they must be identified as not having been included in the original transfer records, someone responsible for sending the information must be identified, and the process of contacting the accepting care team must be completed. If a care team at the accepting hospital identifies these pending tests in review of records, finding the right person at the referring facility to provide the information is a time-consuming and frustrating process. Ultimately, the process of transferring information is unreliable and highly variable.

Finally, providers are only one stakeholder involved in and ultimately not the end beneficiary of the transfer. Patients and their families or decision-makers typically do not participate in the conversations between providers. Because differences may exist between what is discussed between the referring and accepting care teams and the expectations of the family, there may be a misalignment of expectations surrounding the transfer. Sometimes patient or families hope that a transfer will provide a recovery from a diagnosis with a poor overall prognosis, whereas others are not able to be at the patient's bedside if the transfer occurs to a location far from home. The relationship with family is a critical component of providing best patient care, and the transfer process can further complicate that interaction.

The process of transferring a patient between acute care hospitals is complex and variable, factors that increase the risk of being unable to provide optimal care. Standardization and coordination of this process, as has been implemented in many other areas of medical care, may greatly improve the process for patients, surgeons, and hospitals.

EXISTING MODELS OF COORDINATION OF TRANSITIONS OF CARE AS A RESOURCE IMPROVEMENT OF INTERHOSPITAL TRANSFERS

Currently available tools for transitions of care involving interfacility transfers are limited. These tools either do not include transfers from the emergency department,[46] which make up 75% of emergency general surgery transfers at some centers,[28] or focus on critically ill patients.[47] Until frameworks and tools specific to interhospital transfers of surgical patients are more widely available, quality improvement efforts focused on the discharge process may serve as models for improving outcomes among transferred patients and may provide methods to address coordination of care for interhospital transfers. Federal organizations, such as the Institute for Healthcare Improvement and the Centers for Medicare and Medicaid Services, have developed or funded programs for improving care transitions.[18,48] The Agency for Healthcare Research and Quality–funded Reengineered Hospital Discharge Program (Project RED) developed at Boston Medical Center and Boston University resulted in a 30% lower rate of hospital use (rehospitalization and use of the emergency department) within 30 days of discharge. This was accomplished through education about diagnoses, coordination and education about home care and follow-up needs, reviews of the medication plan, expedited dissemination of the discharge summary, provision of a written discharge summary, and a personalized instruction booklet to provide patient education and communicate with the primary care provider. The program also provided for a telephone follow-up including a clinical pharmacist contacting the patient 2 to 4 days after discharge to highlight the recent discussions with the nurse discharge advocate and review medications.[49,50]

Professional societies have also developed various initiatives to improve the transition from hospital to home. The American College of Cardiology developed the Hospital to Home national quality improvement initiative to reduce hospital readmissions and improve the transition to home for individuals who were hospitalized with cardiovascular disease.[51] The program offers a central database of information and strategies focusing on three areas: (1) ensuring a follow-up visit or cardiac rehabilitation referral is in place within a week of discharge, (2) coordinating postdischarge medication management, and (3) education so that the patient can act on signs and symptoms that would require medical attention. In 2009, the American College of Physicians, Society of Hospital Medicine, Society of General Internal Medicine, American Geriatric Society, American College of Emergency Physicians, and the Society for Academic Emergency Medicine addressed gaps in the quality of transitions between inpatient and outpatient settings through a consensus conference.[52] The group established principles and standards for managing such transitions of care.

Models have been developed to conceptualize transitions of care. One of the most high-profile models is the Care Transitions Intervention developed by Coleman and coworkers.[53] This self-management program targets patients with complex medical needs and their caregivers. A transition coach teaches self-management skills focused on (1) medication self-management, (2) use of a dynamic patient-centered personal health record, (3) primary and specialty care follow-up, and (4) an understanding of when to seek help if their medical condition changes. This program resulted in a significant reduction in 30-day (8.3% vs 11.9%) and 90-day (16.7% vs 22.5%) readmission rates and lower hospital costs at 180 days ($2058 vs $2546).

The Transitional Care Model developed by Naylor and coworkers[54] uses a transitional care nurse-led multidisciplinary program for patients older than 70 years that focuses on patient and caregiver understanding, prevention of decline, and medication reconciliation and management. With this transitional care program, patients in the intervention group who were admitted to the medical service had a lower rate of readmission during the first 6 weeks after discharge (10% vs 23%).[55] Application of the principles learned in the development of these care transition programs and modifications of the tools they use could be one avenue to standardize the transfer process and improve the quality of care provided to surgical patients transferred between acute care hospitals.

SUMMARY

We have provided an overview of the challenges faced and opportunity for improvements in ensuring the safety and optimal care of surgical patients who are transferred between hospitals for urgent or emergent care. Ongoing evaluation and research is necessary to further elucidate the reasons that transferred surgical patients fare worse than their peers who are directly admitted. Fortunately, health systems and the stakeholders can seek out the lessons learned from improvements that have been made in the care of patients undergoing other transitions of care to improve the care of patients who are transferred between acute care facilities.

CLINICS CARE POINTS

- Recognize that patients who are transferred between hospitals are at higher risk of poor outcomes than their directly admitted counterparts.
- Be cognizant of the factors that thwart the care of surgical patients who are transferred between hospitals.
- Foster relationships with referring hospitals and providers to ensure continuity of care as patients are moved between facilities.

DISCLOSURE

C. Reinke has nothing to disclose. A. Ingraham has received funding from the Agency for Healthcare Research and Quality (1K08HS025224-01A1) and serves as a Clinical Consultant to the American College of Surgeons for work that is unrelated to the subject of this article.

REFERENCES

1. Beach C, Cheung DS, Apker J, et al. Improving interunit transitions of care between emergency physicians and hospital medicine physicians: a conceptual approach. Acad Emerg Med 2012;19(10):1188–95.
2. Sochet AA, Siems A, Ye G, et al. Standardization of postoperative transitions of care to the pediatric intensive care unit enhances efficiency and handover comprehensiveness. Pediatr Qual Saf 2016;1(2):e004.

3. Bristol AA, Schneider CE, Lin SY, et al. A systematic review of clinical outcomes associated with intrahospital transitions. J Healthc Qual 2019;42(4):175–87.
4. Kind AJH, Smith MA. Documentation of mandated discharge summary components in transitions from acute to subacute care. In: Henriksen K, Battles JB, Keyes MA, et al, editors. Advances in patient safety: new directions and alternative approaches, vol. 2. Rockville (MD): Culture and Redesign); 2008.
5. King BJ, Gilmore-Bykovskyi AL, Roiland RA, et al. The consequences of poor communication during transitions from hospital to skilled nursing facility: a qualitative study. J Am Geriatr Soc 2013;61(7):1095–102.
6. Gilmore-Bykovskyi A, Jensen L, Kind AJ. Development and Implementation of the Coordinated-Transitional Care (C-TraC) Program. Fed Pract 2014;31(2):30–4.
7. Bosk EA, Veinot T, Iwashyna TJ. Which patients and where: a qualitative study of patient transfers from community hospitals. Med Care 2011;49(6):592–8.
8. Kummerow Broman K, Ward MJ, Poulose BK, et al. Surgical transfer decision making: how regional resources are allocated in a regional transfer network. Jt Comm J Qual Patient Saf 2018;44(1):33–42.
9. Hernandez-Boussard T, Davies S, McDonald K, et al. Interhospital facility transfers in the united states: a nationwide outcomes study. J Patient Saf 2017; 13(4):187–91.
10. Reinke CE, Thomason M, Paton L, et al. Emergency general surgery transfers in the United States: a 10-year analysis. J Surg Res 2017;219:128–35.
11. Huntington CR, Cox TC, Blair LJ, et al. Acuity, outcomes, and trends in the transfer of surgical patients: a national study. Surg Endosc 2016;30(4):1301–9.
12. MacKenzie EJ, Rivara FP, Jurkovich GJ, et al. A national evaluation of the effect of trauma-center care on mortality. N Engl J Med 2006;354(4):366–78.
13. Sampalis JS, Denis R, Lavoie A, et al. Trauma care regionalization: a process-outcome evaluation. J Trauma 1999;46(4):565–79 [discussion: 579–81].
14. Shah S, Xian Y, Sheng S, et al. Use, temporal trends, and outcomes of endovascular therapy after interhospital transfer in the United States. Circulation 2019; 139(13):1568–77.
15. Vora AN, Holmes DN, Rokos I, et al. Fibrinolysis use among patients requiring interhospital transfer for ST-segment elevation myocardial infarction care: a report from the US National Cardiovascular Data Registry. JAMA Intern Med 2015; 175(2):207–15.
16. Mehta RH, Stalhandske EJ, McCargar PA, et al. Elderly patients at highest risk with acute myocardial infarction are more frequently transferred from community hospitals to tertiary centers: reality or myth? Am Heart J 1999;138(4 Pt 1):688–95.
17. Rokos IC, Larson DM, Henry TD, et al. Rationale for establishing regional ST-elevation myocardial infarction receiving center (SRC) networks. Am Heart J 2006;152(4):661–7.
18. Ventura T, Brown D, Archibald T, et al. Improving care transitions and reducing hospital readmissions: establishing the evidence for community-based implementation strategies through the care transitions theme. 2010. Available at: www.cfmc.org/integratingcare/files/Care_Transition_Article_Remington_Report_Jan_2010.pdf. Accessed May 10, 2020.
19. Hill AD, Fowler RA, Nathens AB. Impact of interhospital transfer on outcomes for trauma patients: a systematic review. J Trauma 2011;71(6):1885–900 [discussion: 1901].
20. Iwashyna TJ, Kahn JM, Hayward RA, et al. Interhospital transfers among Medicare beneficiaries admitted for acute myocardial infarction at nonrevascularization hospitals. Circ Cardiovasc Qual Outcomes 2010;3(5):468–75.

21. Ingraham A, Wang X, Havlena J, et al. Factors associated with the interhospital transfer of emergency general surgery patients. J Surg Res 2019;240:191–200.
22. Haydar B, Baetzel A, Elliott A, et al. Adverse events during intrahospital transport of critically ill children: a systematic review. Anesth Analg 2020;31(4):1135–45.
23. Singh JM, MacDonald RD, Ahghari M. Critical events during land-based interfacility transport. Ann Emerg Med 2014;64(1):9–15 e12.
24. Singh JM, MacDonald RD, Bronskill SE, et al. Incidence and predictors of critical events during urgent air-medical transport. CMAJ 2009;181(9):579–84.
25. Block EF, Rudloff B, Noon C, et al. Regionalization of surgical services in central Florida: the next step in acute care surgery. J Trauma 2010;69(3):640–3 [discussion: 643–4].
26. Santry H, Kao LS, Shafi S, et al. Pro-con debate on regionalization of emergency general surgery: controversy or common sense? Trauma Surg Acute Care Open 2019;4(1):e000319.
27. Jonasson O, Barrett JA. Transfer of unstable patients: dumping or duty? JAMA 1987;257(11):1519.
28. Philip JL, Saucke MC, Schumacher JR, et al. Characteristics and timing of interhospital transfers of emergency general surgery patients. J Surg Res 2019; 233:8–19.
29. Dy SM, Rubin HR, Lehmann HP. Why do patients and families request transfers to tertiary care? A qualitative study. Soc Sci Med 2005;61(8):1846–53.
30. Misercola B, Sihler K, Douglas M, et al. Transfer of acute care surgery patients in a rural state: a concerning trend. J Surg Res 2016;206(1):168–74.
31. Yelverton S, Rozario N, Matthews BD, et al. Interhospital transfer for emergency general surgery: an independent predictor of mortality. Am J Surg 2018;216(4): 787–92.
32. Santry HP, Janjua S, Chang Y, et al. Interhospital transfers of acute care surgery patients: should care for nontraumatic surgical emergencies be regionalized? World J Surg 2011;35(12):2660–7.
33. Castillo-Angeles M, Jarman MP, Uribe-Leitz T, et al. Risk prediction accuracy differs for transferred and nontransferred emergency general surgery cases in the ACS-NSQIP. J Surg Res 2020;247:364–71.
34. Crippen CJ, Hughes SJ, Chen S, et al. The impact of interhospital transfers on surgical quality metrics for academic medical centers. Am Surg 2014;80(7): 690–5.
35. Holena DN, Mills AM, Carr BG, et al. Transfer status: a risk factor for mortality in patients with necrotizing fasciitis. Surgery 2011;150(3):363–70.
36. Arthur KR, Kelz RR, Mills AM, et al. Interhospital transfer: an independent risk factor for mortality in the surgical intensive care unit. Am Surg 2013;79(9):909–13.
37. Golestanian E, Scruggs JE, Gangnon RE, et al. Effect of interhospital transfer on resource utilization and outcomes at a tertiary care referral center. Crit Care Med 2007;35(6):1470–6.
38. Lucas DJ, Ejaz A, Haut ER, et al. Interhospital transfer and adverse outcomes after general surgery: implications for pay for performance. J Am Coll Surg 2014; 218(3):393–400.
39. Ingraham AM, Jung HS, Liepert AE, et al. Effect of transfer status on outcomes for necrotizing soft tissue infections. J Surg Res 2017;220:372–8.
40. Haley T, Ghaemmaghami V, Loftus T, et al. Trauma: the impact of repeat imaging. Am J Surg 2009;198(6):858–62.
41. Gupta R, Greer SE, Martin ED. Inefficiencies in a rural trauma system: the burden of repeat imaging in interfacility transfers. J Trauma 2010;69(2):253–5.

42. Bertrand J, Fehlmann C, Grosgurin O, et al. Inappropriateness of repeated laboratory and radiological tests for transferred emergency department patients. J Clin Med 2019;8(9):1342.
43. Puls M. Rural surgery - a view from the front lines: "I need to transfer this patient". MD Edge. Surgery; 2018.
44. Harl FNR, Saucke MC, Greenberg CC, et al. Assessing written communication during interhospital transfers of emergency general surgery patients. J Surg Res 2017;214:86–92.
45. Reinke CE, Kelz RR, Baillie CA, et al. Timeliness and quality of surgical discharge summaries after the implementation of an electronic format. Am J Surg 2014; 207(1):7–16.
46. Theobald CN, Choma NN, Ehrenfeld JM, et al. Effect of a handover tool on efficiency of care and mortality for interhospital transfers. J Hosp Med 2017; 12(1):23–8.
47. Malpass HC, Enfield KB, Keim-Malpass J, et al. The interhospital medical intensive care unit transfer instrument facilitates early implementation of critical therapies and is associated with fewer emergent procedures upon arrival. J Intensive Care Med 2015;30(6):351–7.
48. Herndon L, Bones C, Bradke P, Rutherford P. How-to guide: improving transitions from the hospital to skilled nursing facilities to reduce avoidable rehospitalizations 2013. Cambridge, MA.
49. Boston University Medical Center. Project RED (Re-Engineered Discharge). Available at: www.bu.edu/fammed/projectred/index.html. Accessed May 10, 2020.
50. Jack B, Greenwald J, Forsythe S, et al. Developing the Tools to Administer a Comprehensive Hospital Discharge Program: The ReEngineered Discharge (RED) Program. In: Henriksen K, Battles JB, Keyes MA, et al, editors. Advances in Patient Safety: New Directions and Alternative Approaches (Vol. 3: Performance and Tools). 2008. Rockville (MD).
51. Hospital to Home Project. Available at: www.h2hquality.org. Accessed May 10, 2020.
52. Snow V, Beck D, Budnitz T, et al. Transitions of care consensus policy statement American College of Physicians-Society of General Internal Medicine-Society of Hospital Medicine-American Geriatrics Society-American College of Emergency Physicians-Society of Academic Emergency Medicine. J Gen Intern Med 2009; 24(8):971–6.
53. Coleman EA, Parry C, Chalmers S, et al. The care transitions intervention: results of a randomized controlled trial. Arch Intern Med 2006;166(17):1822–8.
54. Naylor M, Brooten D, Jones R, et al. Comprehensive discharge planning for the hospitalized elderly. A randomized clinical trial. Ann Intern Med 1994;120(12): 999–1006.
55. Naylor MD, Brooten D, Campbell R, et al. Comprehensive discharge planning and home follow-up of hospitalized elders: a randomized clinical trial. JAMA 1999;281(7):613–20.

Improving Postoperative Rescue Through a Multifaceted Approach

Amir A. Ghaferi, MD, MS[a],*, Emily E. Wells, MPH[b]

KEYWORDS

- Failure to rescue • Postoperative mortality • Diagnostic error • Patient safety
- Cognitive bias • Clinical decision making

KEY POINTS

- Some of the most effective targets to improve rescue include increasing providers' confidence and competence with earlier recognition and effective management of complications as they develop.
- Developing strategies to strengthen communication and collaboration within interprofessional care teams is also effective.
- Hospital-level factors such as staffing ratios, technology, and teaching status explain only one-third of the variation in hospital rescue rates.
- Safety attitudes, team behaviors, and other organizational culture factors are also drivers of rescue.

INTRODUCTION

Despite more than a decade of safety work in health care, injury and death owing to preventable events remain the third leading cause of death in the United States. Approximately 100,000 Americans die every year after elective inpatient surgery. Wide variation in mortality rates across hospitals suggests substantial opportunities for improvement.[1] Specifically, prior work has identified early recognition of emerging complications and early warning signs of clinical deterioration as primary areas to target.[2] However, there remain significant gaps in our understanding of how to accelerate experiential learning through targeted interventions that improve critical diagnostic and communication skills requisite for detecting and acting on the early stages of clinical decline.

[a] Department of Surgery, University of Michigan, 2800 Plymouth Road, Building 16, 140E, Ann Arbor, MI 48109, USA; [b] Department of Surgery, University of Michigan, 2800 Plymouth Road, Building 16, 167C, Ann Arbor, MI 48109, USA
* Corresponding author.
E-mail address: aghaferi@med.umich.edu
Twitter: @AmirGhaferi (A.A.G.)

Surg Clin N Am 101 (2021) 71–80
https://doi.org/10.1016/j.suc.2020.09.004
0039-6109/21/© 2020 Elsevier Inc. All rights reserved.

surgical.theclinics.com

Although decades of patient safety research have focused on preventing complications in an effort to ultimately decrease mortality, there is growing recognition that high and low mortality hospitals are distinguished less by their complication rates than by how successfully they recognize and manage complications once they occur.[3–6] By appropriately using tools for early recognition and proper treatment, we can combat the system that is propelling failure to rescue (FTR) forward. FTR is defined as death after a major postoperative complication. Successful rescue requires that an optimized structure to communicate exists, to facilitate effective exchanges of information across integrated care teams.

The concept of FTR was first described in 1992 by Jeffrey Silber and collegaues.[7] Over the ensuing 17 years, there were several other papers published describing the phenomenon and establishing associations with hospital structural elements.[8–11] In 2009, a landmark study in the *New England Journal of Medicine* found that, among hospitals participating in the American College of Surgeon's National Surgical Quality Improvement Program, postoperative mortality was not driven by differences in complication rates, but rather FTR. This finding helped to establish FTR as a widely accepted and reported measure. Before this, the Agency for Healthcare Research and Quality had included FTR as one of its Patient Safety Indicators in 2003. Subsequent to the National Surgical Quality Improvement Program study, in 2010 the Centers for Medicare and Medicaid Services began monitoring FTR rates using the Agency for Healthcare Research and Quality Patient Safety Indicator-4 definition and designation. It is also publicly reported on the Centers for Medicare and Medicaid Services Hospital Compare website. There has been some controversy regarding the precise definition of FTR using administrative data, particularly in assessing whether coded complications were potentially present on admission. These have been largely addressed, but, as a result, the National Quality Forum recently removed its endorsement of the Patient Safety Indicator-4 definition of FTR. Nonetheless, the National Surgical Quality Improvement Program and Centers for Medicare and Medicaid Services continue to report this measure giving clinicians, patients, and hospitals the ability to make their own comparisons.

BACKGROUND

Major complications that may develop after surgery—such as blood clots, infections, and heart attacks—are significant causes of death after elective surgery. In recent decades, advances in surgical quality, infection prevention, and other safety measures have decreased postsurgical complications, as well as the deaths that can result from them. However, not all complications are preventable; the unexpected can and does happen after surgery. According to our prior work, we know that hospitals with higher death rates after surgeries do not have higher rates of complications, but do have higher rates of failing to rescue patients who experience them.[1,3] We also know that death rates among patients with major complications also vary widely between hospitals (with as much as an 11-fold difference), and FTR is one of the key drivers of this variation.[4] Therefore, more rapidly identifying and effectively responding to complications when they do occur after surgery presents a major opportunity to improve patient safety and prevent loss of life.[5,12,13] Rescuing a surgical patient is a dynamic process. It requires interpreting and exchanging complex information in moments of crisis among care team members who have different professions and roles.[14]

Our group has used mixed methods over the last decade to understand these specific facets of FTR and developed a 3-pronged approach to improving rescue. We began developing and pilot testing these tools starting in winter 2017 in a large academic hospital in the Midwestern United States. First, we created an expected postoperative course (EPOC) instrument to provide clinicians with a global view of how patients undergoing high-risk procedures progress compared with expected clinical trajectories. Second, we developed an enhanced morbidity and mortality (M&M) case review system (Rescue Improvement Conference or Rescue M&M) that uses the collective experiences of stakeholders from multiple disciplines to identify cognitive bias and implement improvements for the timely treatment of complications. Third, we developed a web-based learning module ("Turning Points") designed to help clinicians identify cognitive bias and enhance diagnostic skill and clinical decision making through real-life postoperative patient scenarios.

Expected Postoperative Course

The first intervention we developed is the EPOC reference tool. This tool was initially constructed around 3 high-risk procedures—cystectomy, pancreaticoduodenectomy, and kidney transplant. Using general care milestones, such as pain control, drain management, diet, ambulation, and respiratory, this instrument follows a patient from postoperative day 0 to discharge. The goal is that, by improving an understanding of normal, this will help clinicians to identify abnormal sooner. In collaboration with unit leadership, we trained nurses to use the EPOC instrument to identify clinical postoperative milestones. This tool was initially intended for use by nurses on a high-acuity surgical unit, but was more widely adopted among advanced practice providers and junior-level house officers who incorporated it into their routine practice.

The development and assessment of the EPOC required several stages of inquiry and refinement. We conducted 16 trend recognition focus groups in summer 2018 where we reviewed clinical scenarios to understand the importance of trends in both normal and abnormal situations. We focused the discussion and learning around common operations and complications and encouraged them to challenge heuristics and create shared mental models. We conducted the focus groups with physician assistants (n = 4), postgraduate year 2 students (n = 3), postgraduate year 6 students (n = 3), and surgical intensive care unit Rapid Response Team (RRT) members (n = 6). During the focus groups, participants commented on the EPOC tool. This feedback can be found in **Table 1**. The Whipple EPOC (**Fig. 1**) was met with the most success. The senior attending surgeon on the service who performs these operations acknowledged that, "The EPOC tool has become a routine part of our daily practice" and "The postpancreaticoduodenectomy milestones have become the standard roadmap of postoperative care." We continue to work toward broader dissemination across hospitals in Michigan.

Rescue Improvement Conference

The second intervention we developed is an enhanced M&M case review system called the Rescue Improvement Conference or Rescue M&M. In fall 2018, we began conducting bimonthly Rescue M&M conferences. This bimonthly conference uses the collective experiences of stakeholders from multiple disciplines to identify and implement multilevel improvements for the timely treatment of complications. This conference is devoted to critically evaluating cases with opportunities for earlier diagnosis of surgical conditions, detection and management of postoperative complications, and/or hospital and team systems-level improvement. The goal is to improve shared mental models and collective vicarious learning among surgical students, residents, and faculty.

We evaluated the impact of these conferences using key stakeholder feedback, including surveys, interviews, and focus groups. Some of the positive feedback we

Table 1
EPOC feedback from trend recognition focus groups

Participants	Quotation
PGY2s (n = 3)	"This sets the expectation so when the patient wakes up and we're not taking their tube out on day one even though their output is really low, they're not afraid that there's something horrifically wrong…it avoids a state of anxiety for the family and explains why the patient looks the way they do."
PGY6s (n = 3)	"One of the biggest driving forces in human learning is pattern recognition. Interns don't have the experience to create pattern recognition, so you have to build in algorithms. I think that's what this is trying to do - build algorithms after looking at patterns of what we've seen and what's expected."
SICU RRT (n = 6)	"I like to check on the patient in bed and see how they look physically. It's more of an inductive process than looking at their vital signs. But as you're looking at their vital signs and you start to get some that are closer to leaving the normal range, then you can try to establish trends to complement this tool."

Abbreviations: PGY, postgraduate year; RRT, registered respiratory therapist; SICU, surgical intensive care unit.

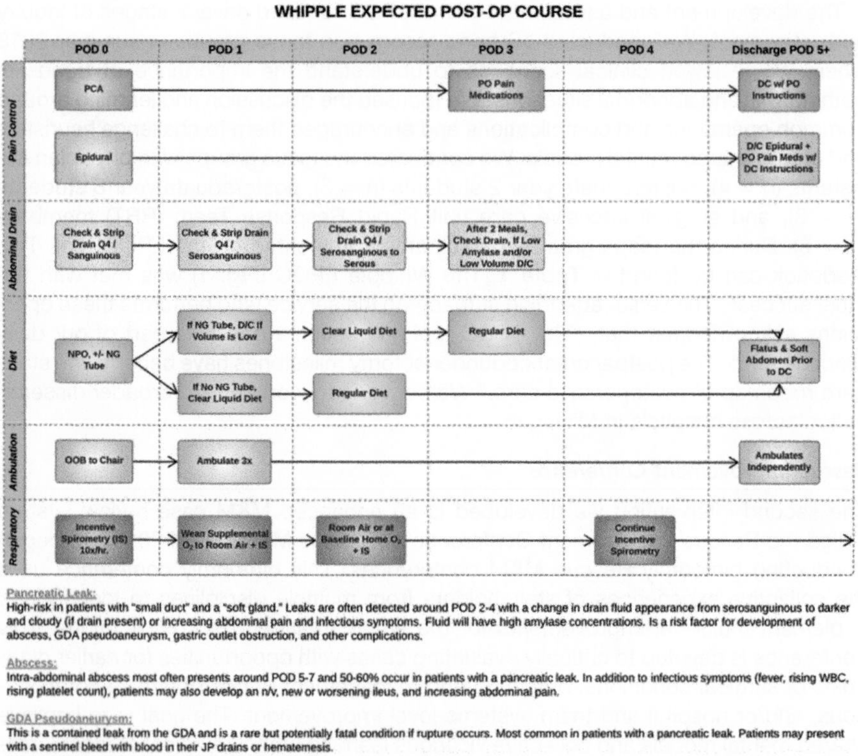

Fig. 1. Example of an EPOC. DC, discharge; D/C, discontinue; GDA, gastroduodenal artery; NG, nasogastric; NPO, nothing by mouth; OOB, out of bed; PCA, patient-controlled analgesia; PO, by mouth; POD, postoperative day.

received included, "This was a tough case with clear issues with bias that would affect every person in a situation like this. It was very useful to hear about every decision point from the people involved, including the trauma team and radiology." Another example was, "Really helpful having representative from other departments at conference. We interface with so many different people, having their input is beneficial for learning and knowing how we can make things better." We have used this feedback to improve Rescue M&M, which has resulted in multiple guideline and protocol changes hospital-wide, and spillover of rescue concepts to regular M&M conferences (see byproducts in **Table 2**). We are also simultaneously developing a repository of key lessons for future use and dissemination.

Additionally, we conducted 12 focus groups and interviews with surgical residents and faculty to collect feedback on Rescue M&M. We interviewed senior and junior residents and attending surgeons. In analyzing the data, we sought to understand how people are "receiving" these conferences. We looked at the positive and negative themes of the conference on learning and rescue improvement. We specifically found that all participants felt that the conferences provided a very different view of morbidity or mortality. Participants felt that often the conference focused less on the clinical nuance of the patient's presentation or the clinical diagnosis, but rather on how the team could have thought differently or how the system could improve to increase the success of rescue. A set of representative quotes from these interviews can be found in **Table 3**. We sought feedback on the differences between Rescue M&M and regular M&M, on effective structure and facilitation approaches, on moderator and resident techniques and skills, on number of cases, on teaching approaches seen at other institutions, on Rescue M&Ms impact on clinical care approaches, and on how content covered during Rescue M&M has been adapted for teaching.

Turning Points

The third intervention we developed is *Turning Points,* an interactive, web-based application that presents brief patient scenarios to introduce and instruct residents on how to identify potential cognitive biases during clinical decision making, and more importantly to enforce strategies to mitigate those biases. Turning Points achieves this through targeted training around anticipated deviations from normal. The module is complication and lesson specific. The goal is to develop shared mental models and to allow front-line clinicians to actively make contingency plans. The conceptual framework for this work was developed by our team and grounded in the principles of high reliability set forth in the organizational management literature.[15,16]

When developing Turning Points, we surveyed house officers to determine what biases to include in the training scenarios. These surveys were conducted during regularly scheduled educational time for our house officers. We received a 100% response rate at each session. We organized biases into 6 categories and provided participants with the name of the bias and its definition. We asked them which biases they were most familiar with, least familiar with, and most interested in learning about. We used their responses to inform case selection to include in the Turning Points module.

With Turning Points, we continue the work to refine and test the tool. We are in the midst of conducting a heuristic evaluation, a think aloud procedure, and performance user testing.[17–19] In a heuristic evaluation, experts critique the content and user interface. In a think-aloud procedure, naïve subjects comment on the program as they use it. In performance user testing, we capture the feasibility, acceptability, and error rates of the application from naïve subjects. As a part of the heuristic evaluation, the research team collaborated with product designers in face-to-face meetings and

Table 2
Examples of change resulting from rescue M&M conference

Topic	Issue	Subsequent Changes to Guidelines and Protocols	Stakeholder Involvement
Bed malfunction	Staff injury and potential patient fall	Modifications to equipment and designation of a clinician responsible for position checks during timeouts and intraoperatively	Patients, house officers, facilities and operations
Fluid management and postoperative AKI prevention or treatment	Lack of standardized I/Os or AKI protocol	Quality improvement action project in surgery by junior residents to standardize I/Os reporting for AKI	AKI patients, surgical residents, faculty
Multifactorial delay in diagnosis	Concerns over the safety of imaging with pregnant patients	Protocol for MRI use vs CT scan use based on week of gestation	Pregnant patients, radiology faculty, emergency department faculty
Accurate preoperative assessment of substance use	Alcohol withdrawal with intensive care unit admission	Standardized use of alcohol withdrawal protocols and guidelines	Patients with alcohol history, surgical residents and faculty

Abbreviations: AKI, acute kidney injury; CT, computed tomography; I/Os, input/output.

Table 3
Rescue M&M resident focus groups and faculty interview data

Participants	Positive Quote	Negative Quote
ADT Residents	"I think the Rescue M&Ms are where the residents feel the most empowered to talk. One of the big positives is getting the resident perspective on things and not attendings being like, "Well, this is the way I would've done it." "In some ways it adds in a little bit of shared language to talk about decision making with attendings or co-residents if you are not seeing eye to eye."	"Any time you're up there [presenting] it's pretty daunting to have to prepare for. I've never had to do it, but I can't imagine it's a thing people look forward to, because it takes a lot of effort to go through a case and know it well enough to do a full 1-h discussion and lead it."
Junior interns	"There are valuable conversations [at Rescue M&M]. There are always 1 or 2 learning points or takeaways that I get from each case, particularly with work-up and management and how to interpret images, which has been valuable." "What works well is the open nature of the conversation, getting feedback through each step of the presentation and the hospital course...the focus on systems level change as opposed to errors in judgment has been valuable for me."	"Thinking about what other players were involved in the complication and having them be involved from the start...so that your whole talk is framed with all those perspectives, not just the surgical side." "It would be helpful to have an orientation session to cover the different types of bias you use or errors that some of the attendings and senior residents think about to give us context."
Attending faculty	"This M&M, because it's not pointing fingers, becomes less about the cognitive stuff...it's an entirely different feel and it lends itself to education and how to better treat things without being shamed...even junior residents can say something without feeling like they're put on the spot." "There's room to discuss issues that are beyond what has become mundane for surgeons - the idea of 'this was a technical error' or 'this was a judgment error' and rather to try and look at things in terms of system-level errors or issues." "[Rescue M&M] allows us to recognize that not all complications are within our control and we can identify things that may be happening repeatedly...there might be a problem that all of us are experiencing...and this is a forum where it's safe to say this has been happening and it's becoming more difficult to manage." "It puts a lot of value on identifying system issues as opposed to individual practices...because that's where the most significant impact for patient care could happen....Rescue M&M advances much more, it touches more people, and more patients."	"This is a small part of a huge hole that doesn't exist right now in terms of stuff that residents don't learn in their time here. Taking care of patients isn't just having medical knowledge. It's understanding the system that you work in, how to utilize it, how to leverage it. So, this is where I think you need to expose trainees more formally through a leadership training or within the curriculum" "There's not enough accountability for the decisions that we're making. In M&M, we focus so much on the patient factors, but a lot of the reasons why we get into these problems is because we are making poor decisions and I don't think that's enough of the focus...This is our time to lay it out there and say, I made a wrong decision, how can I think about this different next time? If we keep saying, it's a system problem or it's a patient problem, then how are we being held accountable for what we do?"

with conference calls over the course of several months. Cases were developed and refined concurrently. As part of the think aloud procedure, approximately 10 surgical trainees (first to third years) will go through the application, with the interviewer asking questions periodically to obtain primarily qualitative feedback. For each page, researchers will ask participants about readability, information sufficiency, clarity and actionability, and organization of the content on the screen. As a part of performance testing (user testing), we will conduct a post-test where at least 12 trainees will assess the feasibility, appropriateness, and acceptability of each scenario.

DISCUSSION

Moving beyond complication prevention and traditional teaching of perioperative care is paramount to improving our surgical outcomes. Increased complexity in the health care system has exacerbated existing inefficiencies in communication and complication detection. The proposed interventions described in this article provide a window into how the field of surgery can move forward with a renewed focus on the education and empowerment of our front-line clinicians. Previous work had focused almost exclusively on macrosystem factors that may affect rescue. Zooming in on the microsystem, namely, the surgical unit and the innumerable interpersonal interactions that take place, is where our novel findings will bring about new change.

As we continue to develop and refine effective tools to improve rescue, we must continue to evaluate where and why failures occur and ultimately implement effective prevention strategies. This process lends itself to potential interventions at the hospital level and even regulatory and certification levels. First, hospitals and health systems should consider implementing quality improvement strategies that increase providers confidence and competence with (1) earlier detection of major complication and (2) effective interprofessional communication of early concerns.[2,14] They should also ensure a culture that prioritizes safety by maximizing staffing strategies (within resource and training constraints), considering nurse to patient ratios and intensivist staffing.[13,20,21] For example, in a study by Ward and colleagues,[22] hospitals with lower FTR rates were more likely to have board certified intensivists; a closed intensive care unit model; overnight in-house surgical coverage; 24/7 inpatient support from hospitalists, advanced practice providers, and residents; and an increased use of rapid response teams compared with hospitals without these resources. Also, in a meta-analysis conducted by Driscoll and colleagues,[23] the analysis found that a higher level of nurse staffing was associated with a decrease in the risk of in-hospital mortality (odds ratio, 0.86; 95% confidence interval, 0.79–0.94). However, no recommendation can be made regarding the optimal nursing ratio required to improve patient outcomes owing to the differences between studies.

Next, regulatory agencies should reevaluate workforce development to provide safe, reliable, and effective care. For example, certification programs across health professions should consider enhancing training requirements that ensure greater exposure to effective rescue scenarios. Professional specialty organizations should consider developing and implementing guidelines to improve rescue and response to crises. Also, they should consider developing networks to share information and best practices on postoperative rescue, including managing specific complications in high-risk groups.

SUMMARY

The work described in this review sheds light on how health care organizations can be engaged to better sense, cope with, and respond to the unexpected and changing demands presented by clinically deteriorating postsurgical patients with life-threatening complications. Also, it will inform further development, testing, and implementation of larger scale rescue-focused initiatives, which could have a direct, population-level impact on reducing mortality in surgical patients. We provide a unique approach to improving rescue across surgical departments. This approach includes using tailored rescue improvement tools and interprofessional learning to enhance staff culture, confidence, and competence with the ultimate focus on decreasing FTR rates.

CLINICS CARE POINTS

- Early recognition and effective communication of patient deterioration are key principles to improve postoperative rescue.
- When seeking to reduce FTR, multifaceted educational and systems approaches to improving diagnostic accuracy is important to train frontline clinicians in prevention.
- Cognitive biases are a root cause of delayed recognition of major complications and can contribute to delayed diagnoses and action taking in deteriorating patients.

DISCLOSURE

This research is funded through grants from the Patient-Centered Outcomes Research Institute (PCORI), the Agency for Healthcare Research and Quality (AHRQ), and the National Institutes of Health (NIH). Dr A.A. Ghaferi also receives salary support from Blue Cross Blue Shield of Michigan as the Director of the Michigan Bariatric Surgery Collaborative.

REFERENCES

1. Ghaferi AA, Birkmeyer JD, Dimick JB. Variation in hospital mortality associated with inpatient surgery. N Engl J Med 2009;361(14):1368–75.
2. Smith ME, Wells EE, Friese CR, et al. Interpersonal And Organizational Dynamics Are Key Drivers Of Failure To Rescue. Health Aff (Millwood) 2018;37(11):1870–6.
3. Ghaferi AA, Birkmeyer JD, Dimick JB. Complications, failure to rescue, and mortality with major inpatient surgery in Medicare patients. Ann Surg 2009;250(6): 1029–34.
4. Ghaferi AA, Birkmeyer JD, Dimick JB. Hospital volume and failure to rescue with high-risk surgery. Med Care 2011;49(12):1076–81.
5. Ghaferi AA, Dimick JB. Variation in mortality after high-risk cancer surgery: failure to rescue. Surg Oncol Clin N Am 2012;21(3):389–95, vii.
6. Sheetz KH, Krell RW, Englesbe MJ, et al. The importance of the first complication: understanding failure to rescue after emergent surgery in the elderly. J Am Coll Surg 2014;219(3):365–70.
7. Silber JH, Williams SV, Krakauer H, et al. Hospital and patient characteristics associated with death after surgery. A study of adverse occurrence and failure to rescue. Med Care 1992;30(7):615–29.
8. Silber JH, Romano PS, Rosen AK, et al. Failure-to-rescue: comparing definitions to measure quality of care. Med Care 2007;45(10):918–25.
9. Aiken LH, Clarke SP, Silber JH, et al. Hospital nurse staffing, education, and patient mortality. LDI Issue Brief 2003;9(2):1–4.

10. Friese CR, Aiken LH. Failure to rescue in the surgical oncology population: implications for nursing and quality improvement. Oncol Nurs Forum 2008;35(5): 779–85.
11. Needleman J, Buerhaus P, Mattke S, et al. Nurse-staffing levels and the quality of care in hospitals. N Engl J Med 2002;346(22):1715–22.
12. Sheetz KH, Waits SA, Krell RW, et al. Improving mortality following emergent surgery in older patients requires focus on complication rescue. Ann Surg 2013; 258(4):614–7 [discussion: 617–8].
13. Ghaferi AA, Dimick JB. Understanding failure to rescue and improving safety culture. Ann Surg 2015;261(5):839–40.
14. McGovern KM, Wells EE, Landstrom GL, et al. Understanding Interpersonal and Organizational Dynamics Among Providers Responding to Crisis. Qual Health Res 2020;30(3):331–40.
15. Ghaferi AA, Myers CG, Sutcliff KM, et al. The Next Wave of Hospital Innovation to Make Patients Safer. Harv Bus Rev 2016. Available at: https://hbr.org/2016/08/the-next-wave-of-hospital-innovation-to-make-patients-safer.
16. Weick KE, Sutcliffe KM. Managing the unexpected : sustained performance in a complex world. Third edition. Hoboken (NJ): John Wiley & Sons, Inc.; 2015.
17. Virzi RA, Sorce JF, Herbert LB. A Comparison of 3 Usability Evaluation Methods - Heuristic, Think-Aloud, and Performance Testing. Designing for diversity, Vols 1 and 2. 1993;37(4):309–13
18. Weiner BJ, Lewis CC, Stanick C, et al. Psychometric assessment of three newly developed implementation outcome measures. Implement Sci 2017;12:102.
19. Ervin JN. An acceptability pilot of the facilitating active management in lung illness with engaged surrogates (FAMILIES) study. Medicine 2020;99(9):e19272.
20. Ghaferi AA, Dimick JB. Importance of teamwork, communication and culture on failure-to-rescue in the elderly. Br J Surg 2016;103(2):e47–51.
21. Myers CG, Lu-Myers Y, Ghaferi AA. Excising the "surgeon ego" to accelerate progress in the culture of surgery. BMJ 2018;363:k4537.
22. Ward ST, Dimick JB, Zhang W, et al. Association Between Hospital Staffing Models and Failure to Rescue. Ann Surg 2018;270:91–4.
23. Driscoll A, Grant MJ, Carroll D, et al. The effect of nurse-to-patient ratios on nurse-sensitive patient outcomes in acute specialist units: a systematic review and meta-analysis. Eur J Cardiovasc Nurs 2018;17(1):6–22.

Provision of Defect-Free Care

Implementation Science in Surgical Patient Safety

Alaina M. Lasinski, MD, Prerna Ladha, MD,
Vanessa P. Ho, MD, MPH*

KEYWORDS

- Implementation science • Implementation research • Dissemination research
- Deimplementation • Implementation frameworks • Implementation strategies

KEY POINTS

- Implementation science is the study of the translation of evidence-based best practices to real-world clinical environments.
- Outcomes of implementation research include acceptability, adoption, appropriateness, feasibility, fidelity, penetration, sustainability, and implementation costs.
- Key frameworks and models introduced, including Translating Evidence into Practice; Consolidated Framework for Implementation Research; Reach, Effectiveness, Adoption, Implementation, and Maintenance; and Expert Recommendations for Implementing Change, that outline domains and strategies to assist researchers identify barriers and facilitate implementation.
- Research methods may include qualitative studies, mixed methods, parallel group, pre-/postintervention, interrupted time series, and cluster or stepped-wedge randomized trials.
- Deimplementation is the study of how to remove outdated, unnecessary, or ineffective practices from the clinical setting and is an equally important component of implementation science.

INTRODUCTION

In today's era of evidence-based medicine, scientific breakthroughs should guide medical care. Unfortunately, it takes approximately 17 years for knowledge gained from research to reach widespread practice.[1] Consequently, patients may receive

Department of Surgery, MetroHealth Medical Center, 2500 MetroHealth Drive, Cleveland, OH 44109, USA
* Corresponding author. Department of Surgery, MetroHealth Medical Center, 2500 Metro-Health Drive, H952, Cleveland, OH 44109
E-mail address: vho@metrohealth.org

Surg Clin N Am 101 (2021) 81–95
https://doi.org/10.1016/j.suc.2020.09.009
0039-6109/21/© 2020 Elsevier Inc. All rights reserved.

surgical.theclinics.com

outdated care for nearly 2 decades. Implementation science (IS) is the study of methods to promote the adoption and integration of evidence-based practices into routine utilization (**Table 1**). IS is the next great global health care research frontier to bridge the crucial gap between knowledge and practice. The World Health Organization identifies the process of implementing proven interventions as one of the greatest challenges facing the global health community.[2]

The goals of this review are to

1. Define implementation science,
2. Discuss key outcomes,
3. Review commonly used frameworks,
4. Describe research methods, and
5. Provide an overview of deimplementation.

Implementation research is typically salient after an intervention is known to be clinically efficacious and effective (**Fig. 1**).[3] In many ways, IS is an extension of familiar processes of clinical efficacy or effectiveness research and quality improvement (QI). Clinical efficacy/effectiveness research aims to establish best clinical practices to improve outcomes at the patient level. With implementation research, however, the best practice is already established, and it focuses on the next steps of improving utilization of effective interventions. Interventions can target policy, organizations, systems, clinical settings such as inpatient floors and outpatient clinics, or providers. QI examines effects of process changes related to health care quality and safety and is typically performed in a local setting. IS research expands on QI principles to allow extrapolation to other settings. IS also includes the study of deimplementation or systematic removal of outdated or low-value care from practice.

IMPLEMENTATION OUTCOMES

Just as clinical research typically examines outcomes such as mortality, key outcomes of IS help researchers to know if an intervention is successful. Proctor and colleagues[4] proposed 8 commonly used and distinct implementation outcomes (**Table 2**):

Table 1	
Implementation science and related research/process definitions	
Type of Research/Process	**Definition**
Clinical effectiveness research	The study of which clinical or public health interventions work best for improving health
Quality improvement	The systematic approach to the analysis of practice patterns to improve performance in health care
Implementation science	The study of the timely uptake of evidence into routine practice; abroad term that includes implementation research, dissemination research, and deimplementation research
Implementation research	The study and use of strategies to integrate best practice, evidence-based interventions into specific settings
Dissemination research	The study of diffusion of materials and information to a particular audience
Deimplementation research	The study of the processes to remove outdated, incorrect, or low-value care from practice

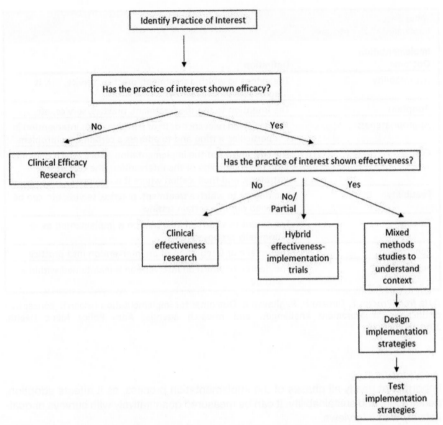

Fig. 1. Process to assist with research efforts. *Adapted from* Lane-Fall MB, Curran GM, Beidas RS. Scoping implementation science for the beginner: locating yourself on the "subway line" of translational research. BMC Med. Res. Methodol. 2019;19(1):133; with permission.

- Acceptability
- Adoption
- Appropriateness
- Feasibility
- Fidelity
- Penetration
- Sustainability
- Cost

These outcomes can be used first as indicators of implementation success, second as indicators of implementation processes, and third as intermediate outcomes in relation to clinical outcomes for effectiveness or quality research.[5]

Acceptability

Acceptability is the belief among stakeholders that a given treatment, process, device, standard, etc. is agreeable or respectable. The complexity and content of the intervention and a stakeholder's familiarity or comfort with it often play a role in that intervention's acceptability. Acceptability is often measured at the stakeholder level and is

Table 2
Implementation outcomes

Implementation Outcome	Definition
Acceptability	The extent to which a treatment, practice, service, etc. is agreeable or satisfactory
Adoption	The intention to use the treatment, practice, service, etc.
Appropriateness	The perceived relevance or fit of a treatment or intervention in a particular setting and to address a certain issue/problem
Cost	The cost impact of the implementation effort, which depends on the complexity of the intervention, the cost of the strategy, and the location where it is deployed
Feasibility	The degree to which a treatment, practice, service, etc. can be carried out in a certain setting
Fidelity	The extent to which an intervention is implemented as originally proposed
Penetration	The uptake or integration of an intervention into practice
Sustainability	The degree to which an intervention is maintained within a setting

Data from Proctor E, Silmere H, Raghavan R. Outcomes for implementation research: conceptual distinctions, measurement challenges, and research agenda. Adm Policy Ment Health. 2011;38(2):65-76.

important at nearly all phases of the implementation process, as it affects adoption, penetration, and sustainability. It can be measured quantitatively with surveys or qualitatively with interviews.

Adoption

Adoption is defined as the decision or action to try to put into effect an intervention or evidence-based practice. It is usually measured at the level of the individual provider or entire organization and is most pertinent at the early to middle stages of implementation, as it refers to the uptake of an intervention into practice. It can be studied with surveys, observation, interviews, or administrative data.

Appropriateness

Appropriateness refers to the believed fit or relevance of an intervention to a given setting and how well it addresses a specific issue or problem. This is different than acceptability in that an intervention may be considered a good fit for a particular audience but may be unacceptable or inappropriate to a provider. Appropriateness is central to the implementation process early, before the adoption phase. It is often analyzed at the level of the individual provider, consumer, or organization and can be studied using surveys, qualitative interviews, or focus groups.

Feasibility

Feasibility is the degree to which an intervention can be implemented within a certain setting.[6] It is important early in the implementation process but is often studied retrospectively as an explanation to why an intervention may have been successful or not. It is analyzed at both the provider and organizational level and is often examined using surveys or administrative data.

Fidelity

Fidelity is defined as the extent to which an intervention was carried out as it was originally intended.[7,8] It is, perhaps, the most commonly studied implementation outcome, as it comments on the integrity to which an evidence-based practice is adhered to through quality of a treatment protocol or adherence to a program. Fidelity represents the achievement of successful translation of treatments from the clinical laboratory to the real-world delivery systems. There are multiple dimensions of fidelity including adherence, quality of delivery, program component differentiation, exposure to the intervention, and participant responsiveness or involvement.[9,10] Fidelity is analyzed at the provider level with observation, ratings, checklists, or self-report and is important at the early to middle stages of the implementation process.

Penetration

Penetration refers to the successful integration of an intervention into a setting or practice. Penetration can be synonymous with "spread" or "reach." An example may include assessing the number of providers who deliver a certain service out of the total number or providers who are expected or qualified to provide the service. It is usually analyzed at the level of the institution in the middle to later stages of the implementation process and can be done with case audits or checklists.

Sustainability

Sustainability is defined as the degree to which an intervention is maintained or integrated throughout a system over time. In order to have successful sustainability, an evidence-based practice may require saturation throughout all levels of an organization. Sustainability is targeted in the later stages of the implementation process and is often studied at the administrator or organizational level. Sustainability can be measured quantitatively with case audits and checklists or subjectively using interviews and questionnaires.

Cost

Cost is the financial implication of an intervention. The cost often depends on the complexity of the intervention, what strategy is used for implementation, and the target setting or location. Cost is analyzed at the provider and institution level and is important at each stage of the implementation process because it affects other outcomes such as adoption, feasibility, penetration, and sustainability. It is often studied with administrative data.

OUTCOME CONSIDERATIONS: TIMELINE, STAKEHOLDERS

Stakeholders and time frames over which the outcome of interest is salient should be carefully considered while planning implementation research. Ideally, the measurement of these outcomes will allow implementation scientists to determine which factors of a treatment or strategy allow for the greatest success of implementation of an intervention over time. For example, fidelity is usually evaluated during initial implementation, whereas adoption can be studied later.[11–14] Feasibility may be important when a new treatment is first used but may be inconsequential once the treatment becomes routine.

Outcomes of interest can be interrelated, can affect each other over time, and can be studied together or sequentially. For example, as an intervention becomes increasingly acceptable within an institution, penetration can increase over time. In this scenario, acceptability may be considered a *leading* indicator or a future predictor of implementation success. A *lagging* indicator such as sustainability may only be observed after the implementation process is mostly complete. Furthermore, the relationship between outcomes can be dynamic and complex. For example, feasibility, appropriateness, and cost will affect an intervention's acceptability. Acceptability will affect adoption, penetration, and sustainability of the intervention.[4] Also, if providers do not have to implement an intervention or treatment with exact fidelity, they may view the intervention as more acceptable.[15]

Depending on the setting, stakeholders can include physicians, patient representatives, nursing staff, administrators, and governmental officials. Stakeholders with varying expertise will bring important perspectives to overcome different barriers. Stakeholders may also value outcomes differently: providers may be most concerned about feasibility, policy makers may be interested in cost, and treatment developers may value fidelity the most. Integrated involvement of key stakeholders throughout the entire planning process is essential to success.

IMPLEMENTATION THEORIES, FRAMEWORKS, AND MODELS

Numerous implementation theories, frameworks, and models exist to help researchers direct and evaluate implementation efforts. Tabak and colleagues[16] identified 61 theories and frameworks and categorized them according to construct flexibility, dissemination and/or implementation activities, and socioecological framework level. Similarly, Nilsen developed a catalog of implementation theories, frameworks, and models but organized them based on 3 aims: (1) describing and/or guiding the process of translating research into practice, (2) understanding and/or explaining what influences implementation outcomes, and (3) evaluating implementation.[17] The frameworks themselves provide a starting point for developing a study design or implementation project by highlighting potential obstacles or catalysts in the actual implementation and dissemination of the research outcomes, especially with regard to how they may need to be adapted to fit local needs. Three commonly used frameworks or models are presented here: Translating Evidence into Practice (TRIP), Consolidated Framework for Implementation Research (CFIR), and Reach, Effectiveness, Adoption, Implementation, and Maintenance (RE-AIM). A catalog of implementation strategies called Expert Recommendations for Implementing Change (ERIC) is also introduced.

Translating Evidence into Practice

TRIP model is an integrated approach to improve the quality and reliability of care that is often used in both QI processes and dissemination research. TRIP has 4 main steps: (1) summarizing the evidence, (2) identifying local barriers to implementation, (3) measuring performance, and (4) ensuring all patients reliably receive the intervention. The fourth step is a circular process involving 4 components: *engagement* of stakeholders to explain why interventions are important; *educating* them by sharing evidence in support of the intervention; *executing* the intervention by designing a toolkit directed toward barriers, implementation, and learning from prior mistakes; and *evaluation* or regular assessment of performance and inadvertent consequences.[18] The model is designed for use in large-scale collaborative projects.

Consolidated Framework for Implementation Research

The CFIR model[19] suggests 5 domains—intervention characteristics (complexity), outer setting (policies or incentives), inner setting (cultural readiness and resources), individual characteristics (knowledge and belief about the intervention), and process (planning)—with multiple constructs under each domain for identifying implementation barriers and facilitators. In addition, CFIR provides a framework to report on the findings of the implementation process and offers sample interview guides to assess each domain. Further information can be found at https://cfirguide.org/.

Reach, Effectiveness, Adoption, Implementation, and Maintenance

RE-AIM is a commonly used implementation science framework developed in 1999 that defines 5 key domains: reach, effectiveness, adoption, implementation, and maintenance.[20,21] Each dimension is an opportunity for intervention, and all dimensions can be addressed within a study. Comprehensive information about the framework and its use is available at their Web site (http://re-aim.org/). The goal of RE-AIM is to allow multidisciplinary stakeholders to pay attention to programmatic elements that will translate into practice. Definitions of each dimension of RE-AIM and key trigger questions to answer for each dimension are presented in **Table 3**.

Expert Recommendations for Implementing Change

The ERIC project used a Delphi method to identify 73 discrete implementation strategies and categorizes them into 9 distinct clusters.[22–24] The strategies are broken down into groups as follows: use evaluative and iterative strategies, provide interactive assistance, adapt and tailor to context, develop stakeholder interrelationships, train and educate stakeholders, support clinicians, engage consumers, and use financial strategies. The ERIC project subsequently defined the relative importance and feasibility of each strategy with the intention of providing knowledge about their perceived applicability and general ratings by experts.[25]

IMPLEMENTATION RESEARCH: HOW TO DO IT
Planning the Study

Implementation studies must be designed appropriately to reflect the outcome of interest and use process-, institution-, or policy-level data outcomes instead of patient-level outcomes. Topics to consider when planning the study include the following:

1. Choosing an appropriate framework and key implementation domains
2. Establishing the intervention target
3. Defining data elements and data sources
4. Involving major stakeholders
5. Addressing anticipated barriers

Some important questions to consider include: how strong are efficacy data? What is the specific implementation barrier being studied, and how should it best be measured? How many settings should be included? How should time-based biases be addressed? What is the internal and external context? What are ideal data sources (prospective data collection, qualitative data, existing medical or administrative data, or a combination)?

Context

Context is the "set of circumstances or unique factors that surround a particular implementation effort" and is a key factor that influences implementation success.[19] For

Table 3
Reach, effectiveness, adoption, implementation, and maintenance dimensions

Dimension	Definition	Key Pragmatic Priorities
Reach	The absolute number, proportion, and representativeness of settings and intervention agents who are willing to initiate a program.	WHO is (was) intended to benefit and who actually participates or is exposed to the intervention?
Effectiveness	The impact of an intervention on important outcomes, including potential negative effects, quality of life, and economic outcomes.	WHAT is (was) the most important benefit you are trying to achieve and what is (was) the likelihood of negative outcomes?
Adoption	The absolute number, proportion, and representativeness of settings and intervention agents who are willing to initiate a program.	WHERE is (was) the program or policy applied and WHO applied it?
Implementation	At the setting level, implementation refers to the intervention agents' fidelity to the various elements of an intervention's protocol. This includes consistency of delivery as intended, adaptations made, and the time and cost of the intervention.	HOW consistently is (was) the program or policy delivered, HOW will (was) it be *adapted*, HOW much will (did) it *cost*, and WHY will (did) the results come about?
Maintenance	The extent to which a program or policy becomes institutionalized or part of the routine organizational practices and policies. Maintenance in the RE-AIM framework also has referents at the individual level. At the individual level, maintenance has been defined as the long-term effects of a program on outcomes after 6 or more months after the most recent intervention contact.	WHEN will (was) the initiative become operational, how long will (was) it be sustained (setting level), and how long are the results sustained (individual level)?

Data from Glasgow RE, Harden SM, Gaglio B et al. RE-AIM planning and evaluation framework: adapting to new science and practice with a 20-year review. Front Public Health. 2019;7:64 and Glasgow RE, Vogt TM, Boles SM. Evaluating the public health impact of health promotion interventions: the RE-AIM framework. Am J Public Health. 1999;89(9):1322-1327.

example, after the introduction of the World Health Organization (WHO) Surgical Safety Checklist across 8 countries worldwide, there was a reduction in morbidity and mortality across all sites but the decline in statistically significant morbidity was only seen at 3 sites and statistically significant mortality at 2 sites.[26] Contextual factors likely affected the implementation process, as well as downstream implementation at other sites, leading to subsequent controversies around the generalizability regarding the overall efficacy of the SCC.[27] Several tools can quantitatively depict contextual factors, such as the Organizational Readiness for Implementing Change tool or the Implementation Climate Scale.[28]

STUDY DESIGNS
Qualitative and Mixed Methods

Qualitative research uses focus groups, interviews, and observations to explain phenomena. *Mixed methods* research thoughtfully uses both quantitative and qualitative research to approach different aspects of a research question. Qualitative studies can be used simultaneously or sequentially with quantitative research and can help researchers understand *how* an intervention functions in specific settings or contexts. Qualitative research performed before quantitative research can help researchers develop mathematically testable hypotheses. Qualitative research can be used after quantitative studies to explain numeric findings or help explain why an intervention succeeded or failed.

Randomized Controlled Trials

Randomized controlled trials (RCTs) are the gold standard to study clinical intervention efficacy. Randomization can occur at the patient-level or at the level of groups (such as a cluster-randomized study). An RCT minimizes bias by spreading confounding variables evenly across groups. RCTs are often costly and time consuming and can be so tightly controlled for internal validity that the findings are not reflective of real-life situations. *Pragmatic RCTs* are designed to occur in real-world settings by removing some restrictions designed to measure efficacy only. RCTs exist along a spectrum of explanatory (higher internal validity) to pragmatic (higher external validity). The PRagmatic-Explanatory Continuum Indicator Summary tool (http://precis-2.org/), designed in 2009 and updated in 2013, can help investigators determine where a trial falls within this spectrum.[29,30]

Alternative Approaches: Parallel Group, Pre-/Postintervention, Interrupted Time Series, Stepped-Wedge

Other study designs have been designed as RCT alternatives. The *parallel group* design randomizes groups to one or more interventions; otherwise the groups are to be treated as similarly as possible. Treatments are allocated randomly, and groups are compared. There are biases inherent to this design, as the groups may be different in unmeasured ways, and temporal factors can affect the treatment and control groups in ways that accentuate or minimize differences.

Pre- and postintervention studies examine data before and after an intervention. These studies are useful for single-center studies where an intervention occurs at a specified time point. A short washout period of noncollection can help allow time for the intervention to take effect. These are subject to time-based biases such as changes in the population over time (eg, influenza in the winter vs the summer), other changes in practice (unrelated interventions that have an effect on the outcome of interest), and increasing knowledge about a topic that occurs concurrently, or even as a result of, the ongoing study. Because of these confounders, it is difficult attribute causation even if statistical effect exists, although these can be feasible for single centers and can provide pilot data for prospective or multicenter studies.

Interrupted time-series (ITS) is a quasi-experimental design that builds on the pre-post concept. ITS use longitudinal data with multiple time points before and after the intervention to examine temporal trends and make causal interpretations.[31] The ITS approach uses multiple time points to assess the preintervention and postintervention effects, allowing for adjustment for temporal trends that existed before the intervention. This methodology can be useful to examine effects after a policy is put into place.

The *stepped-wedge cluster randomized design* is a newer alternative to parallel group designs and require multiple groups (clusters that can be at the level of a nursing floor, hospital, etc).[32] In a stepped-wedge design, interventions are delivered at the cluster level. At the beginning of the trial, none of the clusters receive the intervention (controls). As the trial continues, a randomized cluster or group of clusters crosses to the intervention. At regular intervals, more clusters cross to the intervention, so by the end of the study all clusters are exposed. Each cluster contributes observations from both the control and intervention arms, but the exposure occurs at different times for the cluster, but each center serves as its own control. This methodology removes bias from baseline center-level imbalance. A widespread trend that temporally affects all sites over the study period could be a confounder with this method, but statistical modeling can help adjust for temporal effects.

Limitations and Reporting Quality

As with any newer science, measurement issues can affect the ability to collect and report data. Standardized and validated instruments are not always available, and terminology is not always consistent. Variation in outcome measures can hinder a study's ability to be generalizable and adaptable to other settings. Implementation processes that address one barrier to effectiveness may not overcome a different barrier, so the outcome measure must be chosen correctly to reflect the intervention of interest. Lastly, implementation research assumes an intervention is effective, but if an intervention is not truly effective, an incorrect conclusion may be attributed to an implementation process rather than the intervention itself. As with any other research, the research reporting quality should be held to accepted standards. Reporting guidelines for different study types can be access through the Equator Network (Enhancing the QUAlity and Transparency of health Research, available at https://www.equator-network.org/).

DEIMPLEMENTATION

An indispensable, yet often overlooked component of implementation science is the study of deimplementation. Deimplementation is the discontinuation of interventions that should be stopped because they are (1) harmful or ineffective, (2) not the most efficient or effective, or (3) unnecessary. Although it would be natural to assume that ineffective practices are discontinued when effective practices are discovered, this process is not guaranteed. Intuitively, there are psychological barriers to removing practices that were previously acceptable. In addition, factors such as organizational priorities, cost-benefit analyses, and perceived benefit to the patient can affect both implementation and deimplementation.[33]

Unlearning of old ideas must occur when learning new ideas. Implementation and deimplementation are hence inherently coupled, and transition requires deliberate intellectual and operational effort at an individual and organizational level. One hypothesis is that this coupling allows for the switch to be effort-neutral over time and positively affects change by avoiding overburdening the system when abolishing archaic practices to make room for novel and evidence-based practices.[34] There are 4 types of change by which outdated practices are discarded: partial reversal, complete reversal, reversal with related replacement, and reversal with unrelated replacement.

Partial Reversal

Partial reversal refers to a reduction in the frequency, scale, or breadth of a current outmoded intervention such that it is offered less frequently or to only a subset of the patients for whom it has been most useful. One example from general surgery can be seen with the treatment of severe perforated diverticulitis. Historically, the gold-standard management of perforated diverticulitis was an end colostomy, which subsequently led to a second morbid operation for many patients. Comparable outcomes have been seen with primary anastomoses in selected populations, and practices have evolved such that end colostomy procedures are used more selectively.[35]

Complete Reversal

Deimplementation is a core process of medical evolution. Thankfully, as a result, processes such as "icepick lobotomies" for psychiatric disease and rectal feeding for patients who are *nil per os* are of historical interest only. These are examples of complete reversal, which implies entirely abolishing a certain intervention that has failed to show any benefit for any group of patients in any timespan or circumstance. A more recent example from critical care is that the common practice of routinely changing ventilator circuits was shown to increase the risk of infection and hence is no longer practiced as the standard of care.[36] Complete removal of a practice implies that the practice was not replaced with a better option but simply was no longer used because it was determined to be ineffective or cause harm.

Reversal with Related Replacement

Reversal with related replacement suggests removing an outdated practice while substituting it with one that is closely related but more evidence based or effective. One excellent example of reversal with related replacement is demonstrated by the use of laparoscopy for surgery as new knowledge, skill, and technology became available. Almost 150 years after the open appendectomy was described, laparoscopic appendectomy is now the gold-standard operation for appendicitis.[37]

Reversal with Unrelated Replacement

Reversal with unrelated replacement refers to replacing a practice with one that is different.[38] Currently, some patients with uncomplicated appendicitis do not receive laparoscopic appendectomy but are treated with antibiotics alone, which is an example of unrelated replacement.[39] As another example from trauma surgery, splenectomy was the standard of care for splenic lacerations; however, angioembolization has now replaced surgery as the initial intervention, which allows for both the preservation of the spleen and avoidance of open surgery.[40] Challenges in this type of change are that 2 separate collaborator groups need to be committed to and help facilitate the transition of practice in clinical scenarios.[34]

Widespread lack of deimplementation of outdated therapies contributes to substantial financial waste in the health care system and has a negative impact on patients and organizations. The execution of deimplementation has led to the development of different frameworks to guide the process. A positive feedback loop, or virtuous cycle of deimplementation before implementation, has been described and involves 9 phases: identification of practice for deimplementation, documenting prevalence of current pattern, investigating context and beliefs that maintain the practice, reviewing relevant methods, choosing matched extinction methods, conducting a deimplementation experiment, evaluating consequences, collecting evidence of saved time and resources, and finally, proposing the next practice to be implemented. This framework effectively removes an outdated practice before introducing a new evidence-based one.[41]

Several government policies such as the Choosing Wisely campaign (https://www.choosingwisely.org/), an initiative of the American Board of Internal Medicine, encourages a dialogue between clinicians and patients about which interventions are truly essential, not duplicated, and free from harm. Similarly, the United States Preventative Task Force makes regular recommendations on altering screening modalities and frequencies, with the intention to encourage evidence-based methods and remove those that are no longer best practice.[42]

Deimplementation is increasingly recognized as an important and deliberate component of improving health care delivery. However, in practice, even strong science can be met with implementation resistance due to deep-seated belief in existing treatment paradigms. A recent editorial proposed a framework where evidence-based deimplementation was approached via 3 broad categories: (1) interventions known not to work, (2) interventions where evidence is uncertain, and (3) interventions that are in development where early discussion of evidence can pave the way for eventual deadoption. Deimplementation reflects a commitment to evidence-based practices and deserves greater attention and study, as it is central to the goal of giving patients the best proved therapies.[43]

SUMMARY

Implementation science will be necessary to improve the delivery of care to patients in a systematic and efficient manner, as well as remove unnecessary and ineffective treatments from being used routinely. Understanding the key outcomes of interest, frameworks, and research methods can help researchers effectively perform and communicate implementation findings to bring modern and effective care to all our patients.

CLINICS CARE POINTS

- Use implementation science research methods when a clinical intervention is known to be effective. Implementation research is used to learn about the best way to deliver the intervention to patients.
- When planning an implementation study, ensure that care is taken to discuss barriers to implementation.
- Select your outcome of interest for collection. Commonly used outcomes include: Acceptability, Adoption, Appropriateness, Feasibility, Fidelity, Penetration, Sustainability, Cost.
- Choose a study design and a framework that fits well with your research question.

ACKNOWLEDGMENTS

This publication was made possible by the Clinical and Translational Science Collaborative of Cleveland, KL2TR002547 from the National Center for Advancing Translational Sciences (NCATS) component of the National Institutes of Health and NIH roadmap for Medical Research. Its contents are solely the responsibility of the authors and do not necessarily represent the official views of the NIH.

DISCLOSURES

A.M. Lasinski and P. Ladha have no disclosures. V.P. Ho is supported by the Clinical and Translational Science Collaborative of Cleveland, KL2TR002547 from the National Center for Advancing Translational Sciences (NCATS) component of the National Institutes of Health and NIH roadmap for Medical Research. V.P. Ho spouse is a consultant for Atricure, Sig Medical, Zimmer Biomet, and Medtronic.

REFERENCES

1. Balas EA, Boren SA. Managing clinical knowledge for health care improvement. Yearb Med Inform 2000;(1):65–70.
2. Peters EA, Tran NT, Adam T. Implementation research in health: a practical guide. Alliance for health policy and systems research. Geneva (Switzerland): World Health Organization; 2013.
3. Lane-Fall MB, Curran GM, Beidas RS. Scoping implementation science for the beginner: locating yourself on the "subway line" of translational research. BMC Med Res Methodol 2019;19(1):133.
4. Proctor E, Silmere H, Raghavan R, et al. Outcomes for implementation research: conceptual distinctions, measurement challenges, and research agenda. Adm Policy Ment Health 2011;38(2):65–76.
5. Rosen A, Proctor EK. Distinctions between treatment outcomes and their implications for treatment evaluation. J Consult Clin Psychol 1981;49(3):418–25.
6. Karsh BT. Beyond usability: designing effective technology implementation systems to promote patient safety. Qual Saf Health Care 2004;13(5):388–94.
7. Dusenbury L, Brannigan R, Falco M, et al. A review of research on fidelity of implementation: implications for drug abuse prevention in school settings. Health Educ Res 2003;18(2):237–56.
8. Rabin BA, Brownson RC, Haire-Joshu D, et al. A glossary for dissemination and implementation research in health. J Public Health Manag Pract 2008;14(2):117–23.
9. Carroll C, Patterson M, Wood S, et al. A conceptual framework for implementation fidelity. Implement Sci 2007;2:40.
10. Dane AV, Schneider BH. Program integrity in primary and early secondary prevention: are implementation effects out of control? Clin Psychol Rev 1998;18(1):23–45.
11. Adily A, Westbrook J, Coiera E, et al. Use of on-line evidence databases by Australian public health practitioners. Med Inform Internet Med 2004;29(2):127–36.
12. Cooke M, Mattick RP, Campbell E. A description of the adoption of the 'Fresh start' smoking cessation program by antenatal clinic managers. Aust J Adv Nurs 2000;18(1):13–21.
13. Fischer MA, Vogeli C, Stedman MR, et al. Uptake of electronic prescribing in community-based practices. J Gen Intern Med 2008;23(4):358–63.
14. Waldorff FB, Steenstrup AP, Nielsen B, et al. Diffusion of an e-learning programme among Danish general practitioners: a nation-wide prospective survey. BMC Fam Pract 2008;9:24.
15. Rogers EM. Diffusion of innovations. 5th edition. New York (NY): Free Press; 2003.
16. Tabak RG, Khoong EC, Chambers DA, et al. Bridging research and practice: models for dissemination and implementation research. Am J Prev Med 2012;43(3):337–50.
17. Nilsen P. Making sense of implementation theories, models and frameworks. Implement Sci 2015;10:53.
18. Pronovost PJ, Berenholtz SM, Needham DM. Translating evidence into practice: a model for large scale knowledge translation. BMJ 2008;337:a1714.
19. Damschroder LJ, Aron DC, Keith RE, et al. Fostering implementation of health services research findings into practice: a consolidated framework for advancing implementation science. Implement Sci 2009;4:50.

20. Glasgow RE, Harden SM, Gaglio B, et al. RE-AIM planning and evaluation framework: adapting to new science and practice with a 20-year review. Front Public Health 2019;7:64.

21. Glasgow RE, Vogt TM, Boles SM. Evaluating the public health impact of health promotion interventions: the RE-AIM framework. Am J Public Health 1999;89(9): 1322–7.

22. Powell BJ, McMillen JC, Proctor EK, et al. A compilation of strategies for implementing clinical innovations in health and mental health. Med Care Res Rev 2012;69(2):123–57.

23. Powell BJ, Waltz TJ, Chinman MJ, et al. A refined compilation of implementation strategies: results from the expert recommendations for implementing Change (ERIC) project. Implement Sci 2015;10:21.

24. Waltz TJ, Powell BJ, Chinman MJ, et al. Expert recommendations for implementing change (ERIC): protocol for a mixed methods study. Implement Sci 2014; 9:39.

25. Waltz TJ, Powell BJ, Matthieu MM, et al. Use of concept mapping to characterize relationships among implementation strategies and assess their feasibility and importance: results from the expert recommendations for implementing change (ERIC) study. Implement Sci 2015;10:109.

26. Haynes AB, Weiser TG, Berry WR, et al. A surgical safety checklist to reduce morbidity and mortality in a global population. N Engl J Med 2009;360(5):491–9.

27. Urbach DR, Dimick JB, Haynes AB, et al. Is WHO's surgical safety checklist being hyped? BMJ 2019;366:I4700.

28. Ehrhart MG, Aarons GA, Farahnak LR. Assessing the organizational context for EBP implementation: the development and validity testing of the Implementation Climate Scale (ICS). Implement Sci 2014;9:157.

29. Loudon K, Zwarenstein M, Sullivan F, et al. Making clinical trials more relevant: improving and validating the PRECIS tool for matching trial design decisions to trial purpose. Trials 2013;14:115.

30. Thorpe KE, Zwarenstein M, Oxman AD, et al. A pragmatic-explanatory continuum indicator summary (PRECIS): a tool to help trial designers. CMAJ 2009;180(10): E47–57.

31. Kontopantelis E, Doran T, Springate DA, et al. Regression based quasi-experimental approach when randomisation is not an option: interrupted time series analysis. BMJ 2015;350:h2750.

32. Hemming K, Haines TP, Chilton PJ, et al. The stepped wedge cluster randomised trial: rationale, design, analysis, and reporting. BMJ 2015;350:h391.

33. van Bodegom-Vos L, Davidoff F, Marang-van de Mheen PJ. Implementation and de-implementation: two sides of the same coin? BMJ Qual Saf 2017;26(6): 495–501.

34. Wang V, Maciejewski ML, Helfrich CD, et al. Working smarter not harder: coupling implementation to de-implementation. Healthc (Amst) 2018;6(2):104–7.

35. Acuna SA, Wood T, Chesney TR, et al. Operative strategies for perforated diverticulitis: a systematic review and meta-analysis. Dis Colon Rectum 2018;61(12): 1442–53.

36. Han J, Liu Y. Effect of ventilator circuit changes on ventilator-associated pneumonia: a systematic review and meta-analysis. Respir Care 2010;55(4):467–74.

37. Korndorffer JR Jr, Fellinger E, Reed W. SAGES guideline for laparoscopic appendectomy. Surg Endosc 2010;24(4):757–61.

38. Ho VP, Dicker RA, Haut ER. Dissemination, implementation, and de-implementation: the trauma perspective. Trauma Surg Acute Care Open 2020; 5(1):e000423.

39. Harnoss JC, Zelienka I, Probst P, et al. Antibiotics versus surgical therapy for uncomplicated appendicitis: systematic review and meta-analysis of controlled trials (PROSPERO 2015: CRD42015016882). Ann Surg 2017;265(5):889–900.

40. Stassen NA, Bhullar I, Cheng JD, et al. Selective nonoperative management of blunt splenic injury: an eastern association for the surgery of trauma practice management guideline. J Trauma acute Care Surg 2012;73(5 Suppl 4):S294–300.

41. Davidson KW, Ye S, Mensah GA. Commentary: de-implementation science: a virtuous cycle of ceasing and desisting low-value care before implementing new high value care. Ethn Dis 2017;27(4):463–8.

42. McKay VR, Morshed AB, Brownson RC, et al. Letting go: conceptualizing intervention de-implementation in public health and social service settings. Am J Community Psychol 2018;62(1–2):189–202.

43. Prasad V, Ioannidis JP. Evidence-based de-implementation for contradicted, unproven, and aspiring healthcare practices. Implement Sci 2014;9:1.

Evolution of Risk Calculators and the Dawn of Artificial Intelligence in Predicting Patient Complications

Jerica L. Podrat, MD[a], Fernando Ramirez Del Val, MD, MPH[a],
Kevin Y. Pei, MD, MHSEd[b],*

KEYWORDS

- Artificial intelligence • Morbidity • Risk calculator

KEY POINTS

- Risk calculators are tools to help surgeons conceptualize and discuss surgical risk.
- Risk calculators have evolved in complexity to be patient and procedure-specific.
- Artificial intelligence algorithms can sift through vast volumes of data to simplify risk assessment for the surgeon.
- The incorporation of artificial intelligence algorithms into electronic medical records is an ongoing area of study.

INTRODUCTION

There is considerable uncertainty in health care and risk prediction plays a pivotal role in our surgical community's ability to drive clinical decisions, counsel patients, and evaluate outcomes. Studies have shown that clinicians are imperfect when predicting medical and surgical risk and often rely on the gestalt of practice experience and global assessment of patient status.[1–3] Surgical risk calculators (RCs) are a set of tools with the potential to mitigate the highly variable perception of patient risk. RCs are increasingly used to assess the likelihood of complications and mortality in the immediate postoperative period. Classically, perioperative risk was determined by the combined intuitions of the participating surgeon and anesthetist.[4]

Although the American College of Surgeons National Surgical Quality Improvement Program (ACS NSQIP) is ubiquitous at the time of this writing, it was not always this

[a] Department of Surgery, Houston Methodist Hospital, 6550 Fannin Street, Suite SM1661, Houston, TX 77030, USA; [b] Parkview Health GME, 2200 Randallia Drive, Administration, Fort Wayne, IN 46805, USA
* Corresponding author.
E-mail address: kevin.pei@parkview.com

Surg Clin N Am 101 (2021) 97–107
https://doi.org/10.1016/j.suc.2020.08.012
0039-6109/21/© 2020 Elsevier Inc. All rights reserved.

way. The need for better accountability in medicine was highlighted in the 1980s by the predecessor of the Centers for Medicare and Medicaid Services, the Health Care Financing Administration, through the publication of hospital-level mortality data.[5] This early attempt for transparency and depiction of surgical risk was unfortunately not adjusted to patients' comorbidities and was therefore deemed to be biased and difficult to interpret. In turn, the earliest iteration of the surgical standard for RCs, The Society of Thoracic Surgeons (STS) Adult Cardiac Risk Model, was published.[6] In it, The STS identified 25 and 10 variables through univariate and multivariate analysis, respectively, that influenced operative mortality.

Similar initiatives to better understand patient care performance followed with the creation of the Veteran Affairs National Quality Improvement Program in the mid-1980s, which ultimately resulted in the creation of the NSQIP in 1994, allowing for risk-adjusted comparisons of outcomes between 133 Veteran Affairs hospitals[7,8] and served as a model for the ACS NSQIP.

As surgeries evolve in complexity and the practice of evidence-based medicine becomes more important, preoperative and corresponding postoperative data points are being used to better assess patient risk and operative outcomes. Medical decision making continues to lean toward patient-centered care and patients have a greater role in this process. We have relinquished paternalistic medicine, instead choosing to empower our patients with data and statistics. This process further highlights the importance of risk prediction models. With the availability of big data,[9] the focus on patient-centered care coalesces in the development of precision surgery, necessitating the development and use of tools that can facilitate these conversations.

Multiple RCs have been proposed, developed, and validated (**Fig. 1**), all incorporating varying levels of data. Development and validation require the collection of multiple large volumes of high-quality data that represent the population of interest. These data points can then be used to design an algorithm to predict a given risk for a

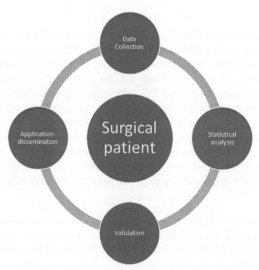

Fig. 1. Representation of the cyclic nature of RC development, validation, and use. The surgical patient is at the center of the chart. Data collection is the basis of the RC, and these data undergo statistical analysis. This analysis leads to an RC, which then undergoes validation. The validated RC can then be applied to the patient. However, continued data collection and revalidation are essential for RC maintenance and accuracy.

determined intervention or condition, yielding an RC. The RC is then validated using different datasets from the one used in the creation of the algorithm, but which are also representative of the population of interest.[10]

The most widespread method to create RCs has been the use of regression models; logistic and hazards models yield odds ratios and hazard risks, respectively. Early iterations of these algorithms suffered from the introduction of considerable selection bias because systematic approaches to their development were less prevalent. The introduction of automated processes like stepwise, backward, and bidirectional elimination has resulted in more objective models as long as adequate validation techniques are used.[11] Although various methods exist to determine the model's accuracy, in logistic regression models the use of the c-statistic is standard. These traditional statistical methods to analyze data and produce risk models have several limitations. Of particular importance are difficulties in dealing with large volume and nonlinear data, which in turn limit their use in finding cluster associations.

To better illustrate the use, prevalence, and limitations or RCs, we describe commonly used calculators, including the American Society of Anesthesiologists Physical State Classification (ASA-PS), the Acute Physiology and Chronic Health Evaluation II (APACHE II), the Physiologic and Operative Severity Score for the enumeration of Morbidity and mortality (POSSUM) and the modified version, Portsmouth POSSUM (P-POSSUM), ACS NSQIP Surgical Risk Calculator (SRC), and the STS Risk Model. We will also discuss the most common hindrances to the use of RCs in daily use. Finally, we will touch on how artificial intelligence (AI) models have been designed to alter the way we look at risk assessment and the current challenges to RC widespread use.

EXAMPLES OF COMMONLY USED RISK CALCULATORS

The ASA-PS is a preoperative risk assessment tool developed in 1940 by the American Society of Anesthetists and one of the most widely used disease severity classification systems.[1,3] It has since undergone multiple revisions and to date includes 6 categories, referred to as Physical States (PS) based on the burden of systemic disease (Table 1).

There are several studies assessing the validity of the ASA-PS based on the user, including anesthesiologists, surgeons, and medical physicians, and the validity of their assessment.[12,13] The ASA-PS effectively stratifies surgical patients into increasing risk groups but fails to consider aggregated risk in patients with multiple comorbidities. Via prospective data, Wolters and colleagues[14] suggested that although the ASA-PS is an adequate predictor of postoperative outcome and can aid in preoperative optimization, it must be combined with perioperative variables such as intraoperative blood loss and duration of ventilatory support as well as need for and duration of the intensive care unit (ICU) stay. Additionally, the ASA-PS does not incorporate the type of surgical procedure and therefore does not assess individualized or procedure-specific risk.[15] Anecdotally, there can also be some subjectivity in a clinician's perception of physical states. Although widely used both in clinical practice and research, its design is for risk stratification and global postoperative assessment. Accordingly, the ASA-PS lacks the granularity or ability to predict specific postoperative outcomes.

A common, nonsurgical RC is the APACHE, which was designed to assess 30-day mortality in ICU patients.[16] Developed in the 1970s, it requires large volumes of weighted data and computational bandwidth to generate risk analysis. Because of the unwieldy nature of APACHE, APACHE II was designed in 1985 to be more user friendly.[17] Data points for APACHE II include a history of organ failure or

Table 1 ASA-PS classification		
Physical State (PS)	**Criteria**	**Examples**
PS1	Healthy patient with no exercise tolerance limitations	Healthy patient, no past medical history
PS2	Mild systemic disease, well-controlled	Well-controlled hypertension or diabetes
PS3	Severe systemic disease with some functional limitation	Poorly controlled hypertension or diabetes
PS4	Severe systemic disease that is a constant threat to daily life, that is, poorly controlled or end-stage disease	End-stage renal disease without routine dialysis, severe cardiac dysfunction
PS5	Moribund patient, not expected to survive without surgery within 24 hours	Mesenteric or bowel ischemia in a patient with severe cardiac dysfunction
PS6	Declared brain dead	

Based on ASA Physical Status Classification System 2019 of the American Society of Anesthesiologists. A copy of the full text can be obtained from ASA, 1061 American Lane Schaumburg, IL 60173-4973 or online at http://www.asahq.org.

immunocompromise, age, vital signs, oxygen requirement, renal status, Glasgow Coma Scale, and pH.[17] APACHE II was designed to use the worst parameters within the last 24 hours for patients newly admitted to the ICU, and not transferred from other units.[17] Although not its original purpose, APACHE II has been used for perioperative risk assessment.[18] Oliver and colleagues[18] generated a meta-analysis looking at validation, discrimination, and calibration of the most common RCs used before emergency laparotomy. They found that, when applied to heterogeneous populations undergoing emergency general surgery, the APACHE II was able to differentiate between 30-day mortality and survival well (area under the curve 0.76–0.098) and had the most consistent accuracy of RCs analyzed. Of note, they found that several institutions used APACHE II as their only preoperative RC.

POSSUM and the modified version, the P-POSSUM, is another commonly used surgical RC. POSSUM was originally described in 1991 and uses 62 data points, of these 48 are physiologic (including cardiac, respiratory, and renal function, as well as the presence of malignancy) and 14 are surgical (including the number of surgeries, types of surgery, and blood loss). POSSUM has been found to overestimate mortality by more than double.[19,20] In 1998, this calculator was decreased to a validated 18 data points, 12 physiologic and 6 surgical to better predict mortality.[15,21] Scott and colleagues[15] evaluated the validity of POSSUM and P-POSSUM against more recent data from patients who underwent surgery between 2000 and 2008. The authors found that although the POSSUM and P-POSSUM are able to differentiate between survivors and nonsurvivors, they were poor estimators of mortality, underestimating mortality risk across surgical specialties.[15]

The ACS NSQIP is an initiative by more than 700 hospitals in the United States to collect standardized preoperative and postoperative data.[22] The NSQIP SRC was developed in 2013 with data from 343 NSQIP participating institutions comprising 1,414,006 patients and 1557 unique Current Procedural Terminology codes to assess universal and procedure-specific risk. The SRC uses the input of 21 data points, including the specific procedure and ASA classification. NSQIP SRC has been assessed against comparable universal and procedure-specific RCs and has been shown to have similar mortality and complication predictive capacity.[22]

The first iteration of the STS Risk Model was done in 1994[23] and used Bayesian statistics to analyze data from the recently created STS database.[24] As the database from which the risk model was created increased in data collection points, the risk model grew in complexity. Expanding from its focus on 1 procedure (coronary artery bypass grafting) to include most adult cardiothoracic surgeries for multiple end points such as length of stay, complications, and operative mortality. A signature characteristic of the STS risk model is the recalibration of the expected number of events to meet the observed number of events, yielding an observed to expected number of events ratio of 1, which can be used to assess performance across different patient and provider strata. The risk model has been used to set a default number of variables for research purposes using the STS database, to asses performance (at a geographic, hospital-wide, or individual level), and to establish a baseline risk for shared decision making during physician-patient counseling. It is one of the most robust prediction models in surgery, and the STS database has become the gold standard for prospectively collected clinical data.

LIMITATIONS OF CURRENT SURGICAL RISK CALCULATORS

Although RCs serve as valuable tools for the surgeon, anesthesiologist, and the patient, they have limitations. All RCs are limited in their generalizability based on input data, including patient population, geographic region, and follow-up interval.[10] The creation of new RCs is limited by the manpower required for extensive data collection and input, difficulty with dissemination to the scientific community, and the requirement for regular recalibration based on new data. The development of risk models requires careful methodology. Consideration of the development of parsimonious versus nonparsimonious models, end point selection, target procedures, interaction terms, and collinearity. With any large database, there may be inherent biases despite mitigation strategies. For example, in 1 common end-of-life surgical discussion, a patient is advised that there is a certain percentage of complication and death. However, because the ACS-NSQIP database only contains data from patients undergoing an operation, we are unable to counsel the patient as to how the percentages of complications and death change without surgery. The clinician and researcher must be particularly mindful of whether the prediction model is suitable in any particular scenario.

The ASA-PS uses a single, broad variable and can only provide generalizable risk. It is not specific to the cumulative patient risks, nor to the procedure. POSSUM and P-POSSUM are limited in predicting mortality. APACHE II was not intended for use outside of the ICU, and although it serves as a good estimate of mortality, it is not procedure specific. Similarly, the STS risk model has several limitations, including coverage of infrequent procedures. It is also unable to capture the risk of covariates that confer considerable perioperative risk but are not included in the data analysis, like chest radiation, destruction of myocardial tissue in patients with endocarditis, and markers of patient frailty. The NSQIP SRC, despite its vast volume of data, was developed using only 10% of surgical patients and procedures that occur in the United States annually, whereas NSQIP itself comprises 30% of all surgical patients. The APACHE II requires 12 data points, POSSUM requires 18, and the NSQIP SRC suggests but does not require 21, with the caveat that more variables give a more precise assessment of risk.[18]

Another limit of RC development is cost. The RCs described elsewhere in this article were developed in the United States, a nation of wealth. In juxtaposition to this, the African Surgical Outcomes Study was developed using the prospective risk and outcome data of 11,422 patients from 247 hospitals in more than 25 countries in Africa; more than 1000 health care workers participated in the data collection.[25] However, this initial investment is not the end of RC development; as practice changes, recalibration and subsequent revalidation of RCs become essential for continued accuracy and precision. In 2016, Liu and colleagues[26] found that after recalibration, the NSQIP SRC outperformed the nonrecalibrated SRC in estimating patient risk for low, medium, and high-risk procedures. This illustrates that for RCs to maintain efficacy, there must be thorough, timely, and continuous interrogation and validation.

Physician-reported data suggest that RCs are not frequently used in practice by physicians and residents.[27,28] To assess the effect of RCs on surgical decision making, Sacks and colleagues[27] invited all general surgeons in ACS who had completed or were currently in residency to complete a survey and series of vignettes in 2014. Using hypothetical vignettes (surgical emergencies including mesenteric ischemia, gastrointestinal bleed, small bowel obstruction, and acute appendicitis), one-half with NSQIP RC data and one-half without, the authors asked participating surgeons to assess the risk to the patient and make treatment recommendations. The goal was to ascertain the impact of RC data on the assessment of risk and ultimately on surgical decision making. Surgeons who completed the vignettes without NSQIP data assessed the patients to have higher surgical risk than the NSQIP data suggest. However, surgeons in the intervention group assessed the same vignette patients as having a lower surgical risk. Sacks and colleagues showed that having RC data altered physician assessment of risk, but ultimately did not significantly alter the surgical intervention recommendations. The authors also recognize limitations to their study, noting that hypothetical vignettes and analysis do not adequately consider aspects of real-time medical care, particularly when applied to emergency surgical cases such as those used in their chosen vignettes.

In a complementary study, Leeds and colleagues[28] sent a survey to 320 US-based general surgery residents across 4 institutions. Only 26% of responders reported using a risk communication strategy other than direct verbal communication and sketch diagrams; 17% of responders reported using RCs more than 50% of the time in risk communication. The authors suggest that a lack of familiarity, exposure, and training that incorporates RCs are at the root of their lack of use by surgical trainees. They also suggest that the incorporation of RC data analysis into the EMR would allow for a more user-friendly addition to daily practice. In this way, assessment of risk would not add to current workflows and ultimately allow for seamless use in practice.

ARTIFICIAL INTELLIGENCE MODELS

The development of big databases has posed unique challenges. Traditional statistical methods are unable to perform timely analysis of these datasets. There is also a suggestion that Bayesian statistics oversimplifies the complexity of physiologic interaction in risk/outcome predictions. These limitations of traditional analysis have fueled advances in AI. AI modeling, which includes machine learning, deep learning, and cognitive computing, has the potential to mine big data, improve patient care, and potentially further our understanding of rare or heterogeneous disease process, furthering the goal of precision medicine.[29] Furthermore, the use of AI in risk assessment could result in real-time tools to support clinical decisions using data from multiple electronic medical records.[30] This could aid in the current over/underestimation of risk stratification models in different patient populations.

Machine Learning

Machine learning is a repertoire of techniques that use big data to solve complex problems by recognition of interaction patterns among variables.[31] An in depth analysis of AI is beyond the scope of this context, but we provide a brief overview. It can be categorized into 3 subtypes. The first is supervised learning, best used for regression and classification problems, and requires that a human place labels on the dataset before the algorithm is run. This type of machine learning can be used in pattern recognition within a limited number of diagnoses to automate the interpretation of images, electrocardiograms, and laboratory values.[32] It has also been used in the development of multiple risk models, including the development of predicting scores for embolic events in atrial fibrillation using data from the Framingham study.[33] This are is perhaps one of greatest promise because it is not only able to make risk assessments that are evident to clinicians, but it is also able to discover new hidden relations.

The second type is unsupervised learning, which identifies novel and naturally occurring associations from hidden patterns without human feedback. Interest in these types of algorithms spawns from the effort to redefine heterogenous multifactorial disease processes to better resemble their pathophysiology and identify new treatment strategies. A downside of unsupervised machine learning is that its results are more difficult to interpret, compared with other types of machine learning.[34] The third type, reinforcement learning, is a mixture of supervised and unsupervised learning. All 3 types identify errors (with or without preestablished labels) to optimize the accuracy of the algorithms. There are multiple algorithms within each type of machine learning, which are better used in different circumstances depending on the outcome of interest, the type of database, training time, learning curve, and the number of parameters. In contrast to traditional statistical analysis methods, these algorithms work with nonlinear relations, are more flexible, and outperform the predictive accuracy of logistic regression models.

Deep Learning

Deep learning is a type of machine learning that uses multiple layers of networks. Inspired by the human brain's network of neurons, deep learning generates predictors from raw input with no limitation in working memory. It works well with noisy data and has been used in image pattern recognition with great results. However, it requires exceedingly large datasets and deep-learning–capable machines. Deep learning has already been shown to outperform different types of regression models in predictive models for opioid overdose risk in patients with opioid prescriptions.[35] However, because deep learning uses multiple layers it is susceptible to producing overfitted models.

Last, cognitive imputing mimics the human thought process of self-learning systems through machine learning, natural language processing, and pattern recognition. Its best-known example is IBM Watson, who has won the game of *Jeopardy* and has been used to optimize care for patients with lung cancer.

Examples of Artificial Intelligence in Medicine

The development of AI continues to expand and in health care, AI is applicable in multiple aspects of health care.[36,37] AI has been used to develop predictive algorithms for drug use, cancer survival, and postoperative complications. In a cohort of more than 500,000 Medicare beneficiaries, a deep neural network was able to better identify risks for opioid overdose using administrative data when compared with multivariate logistic regression, least absolute shrinkage and selection operator-type regression, random forest, and gradient boost machine (C-statistic = 0.9 and a sensitivity of 92% with a specificity of 75% for the deep neural network).[35]

A direct comparison of risk-predictive models in surgical patients has yielded encouraging results. In 2016, Thottakkara and colleagues[38] compared the performance of risk predictive models for postoperative sepsis and acute kidney injury. Using data from more than 50,000 adult surgical patients, they showed good performance for generalized additive models and support vector machines compared with logistic regression and naïve Bayes classifiers. An advantage of generalized additive models in this study was their ability to account for nonlinear relations in continuous variables (age, glomerular filtration rate, and hematocrit), a limitation in regression model analysis.

Risk factors for long-term survival in patients with cancer have long been a principal focus on research, because they not only help to set expectations, but also provide insight into patient characteristics that may benefit less or more from various interventions. Recently, Karadaghy and associates[39] from the University of Kansas developed a 5-year survival predictive model for patients with oral squamous cell carcinoma using machine learning. Its importance, over traditional oncologic survival models, lies in its ability to develop absolute risk estimates for individual patients, which in turn can be used to offer personalized patient care by going beyond the influence of the TNM staging and into patients' demographic, treatment, and pathologic variables.

There have been several attempts to incorporate AI into electronic medical record (EMR) systems.[40,41] Bihorac and colleagues[40] are such an example, and developed and validated a surgical risk algorithm that uses machine learning and is designed to be compatible with any EMR. The goals of the authors were for it to be fully automated, to successfully predict the probability of 8 postoperative complications (infectious and mechanical wound complications, acute kidney injury, mechanical ventilation, ICU admission for more than 48 hours, cardiovascular complications, neurologic complications and/or delirium, sepsis, and venous thromboembolism), and to calculate risk probabilities for death at varying time intervals after the index surgery. Input data is routinely found in the EMR and includes:

- Admission type (medical or surgical)
- Weekday versus weekend admission
- Zip code (demographic information, social determinants of health)
- Time of surgery from admission
- Number of diagnoses
- Basic laboratory data (basic metabolic panel, complete metabolic panel, complete blood count, urinalysis)
- Medications on admission (antibiotics, vasopressors, nephrotoxic medications, nonsteroidal anti-inflammatory drugs)
- Past medical history (congestive heart failure, peripheral vascular disease, hypertension, chronic kidney disease, end-stage renal disease, obesity, weight loss, fluid and electrolyte disorders, diabetes, cancer, liver disease)

The authors note that limitations are similar to already established RCs, including data bias based on the input population dataset necessitating retraining and validation with additional datasets to improve generalizability. Coding data was used in the algorithm to find complications in patient's EMRs, and these also require frequent reevaluation.

SUMMARY

Physicians face an ever-growing need for improved assessment and communication of surgical risk. Addressing this need starts with RCs themselves and the evolution of procedure and patient-specific RCs such as the NSQIP SRC and STS. These tools are not without limitation, requiring continual maintenance and thorough interrogation for continued accuracy. There is also the issue of dissemination; RCs are not widely used by surgical residents or attendings per self-reported studies. Implementing RCs use into daily practice can be a hindrance to current workflows and may not influence patient care. With the incorporation of AI, assessment of risk can be automated, allowing for ease of use and therefore increasing use of formal risk assessment, but this is a field in its nascent stage and requires further study. The ultimate goal of the implementation of AI into health care is to predict outcomes, not just the assessment of risk. Furthermore, its applications can span into utility cost reduction, the development of precision medicine for diagnostic and treatment purposes, minimizing overuse of resources, and incorporation of best care practices.

CLINICS CARE POINTS

- Surgical RCs are tools for the assessment of complications and mortality in the immediate postoperative period.
- Surgical RCs have changed over time to encompass more data and therefore become more generalizable.
- Current trends demand that RCs confer procedure and patient-specific risk assessment.
- The collection of large volumes of data is an essential part of RC development.
- AI can ease the burden of data mining and allow for more rapid, automated risk assessment.

DISCLOSURE

The authors have nothing to disclose.

REFERENCES

1. Healy JM, Davis KA, Pei KY. Comparison of internal medicine and general surgery residents' assessments of risk of postsurgical complications in surgically complex patients. JAMA Surg 2018;153(3):203–7.
2. McDermott R. Medical decision making: lessons from psychology. Urol Oncol 2008;26(6):665–8.
3. Sjoberg L. Factors in risk perception. Risk Anal 2000;20(1):1–11.
4. Chand M, Armstrong T, Britton G, et al. How and why do we measure surgical risk? J R Soc Med 2007;100(11):508–12.
5. Fleming ST, Hicks LL, Bailey RC. Interpreting the health care financing administration's mortality statistics. Med Care 1995;33(2):186–201.
6. Kouchoukos NT, Ebert PA, Grover FL, et al. Report of the Ad Hoc Committee on risk factors for coronary artery bypass surgery. Ann Thorac Surg 1988;45(3):348–9.
7. Fuchshuber PR, Greif W, Tidwell CR, et al. The power of the National Surgical Quality Improvement Program–achieving a zero pneumonia rate in general surgery patients. Perm J 2012;16(1):39–45.

8. Massarweh NN, Kaji AH, Itani KMF. Practical guide to surgical data sets: Veterans Affairs Surgical Quality Improvement Program (VASQIP). JAMA Surg 2018; 153(8):768–9.

9. Cobb AN, Benjamin AJ, Huang ES, et al. Big data: more than big data sets. Surgery 2018;164(4):640–2.

10. Mansmann U, Rieger A, Strahwald B, et al. Risk calculators-methods, development, implementation, and validation. Int J Colorectal Dis 2016;31(6):1111–6.

11. Edwards AL. Multiple regression and the analysis of variance and covariance. Multiple regression and the analysis of variance and covariance. New York: W H Freeman/Times Books/Henry Holt & Co; 1985. p. xv, 221.

12. Abouleish AE, Leib ML, Cohen NH. ASA provides examples to each ASA physical status class. ASA Newsl 2015;79(6):38–49.

13. Owens WD, Felts JA, Spitznagel EL Jr. ASA physical status classifications: a study of consistency of ratings. Anesthesiology 1978;49(4):239–43.

14. Wolters U, Wolf T, Stützer H, et al. ASA classification and perioperative variables as predictors of postoperative outcome. Br J Anaesth 1996;77(2):217–22.

15. Scott S, Lund JN, Gold S, et al. An evaluation of POSSUM and P-POSSUM scoring in predicting post-operative mortality in a level 1 critical care setting. BMC Anesthesiol 2014;14(1):104.

16. Knaus WA, Zimmerman JE, Wagner DP, et al. APACHE-acute physiology and chronic health evaluation: a physiologically based classification system. Crit Care Med 1981;9(8):591–7.

17. Knaus WA, Draper EA, Wagner DP, et al. APACHE II: a severity of disease classification system. Crit Care Med 1985;13(10):818–29.

18. Oliver CM, Walker E, Giannaris S, et al. Risk assessment tools validated for patients undergoing emergency laparotomy: a systematic review. Br J Anaesth 2015;115(6):849–60.

19. Copeland GP, Jones D, Walters M. POSSUM: a scoring system for surgical audit. Br J Surg 1991;78(3):355–60.

20. Prytherch DR, Whiteley MS, Higgins B, et al. POSSUM and Portsmouth POSSUM for predicting mortality. Physiological and Operative Severity Score for the enUmeration of Mortality and morbidity. Br J Surg 1998;85(9):1217–20.

21. Carvalho ECME, DE-Queiroz FL, Martins-DA-Costa BX, et al. The applicability of POSSUM and P-POSSUM scores as predictors of morbidity and mortality in colorectal surgery. Rev Col Bras Cir 2018;45(1):e1347.

22. Bilimoria KY, Liu Y, Paruch JL, et al. Development and evaluation of the universal ACS NSQIP surgical risk calculator: a decision aid and informed consent tool for patients and surgeons. J Am Coll Surg 2013;217(5):833–42.e1-3.

23. Edwards FH, Clark RE, Schwartz M. Coronary artery bypass grafting: The Society of Thoracic Surgeons National Database experience. Ann Thorac Surg 1994; 57(1):12–9.

24. Shahian DM, Jacobs JP, Badhwar V, et al. The Society of Thoracic Surgeons 2018 adult cardiac surgery risk models: part 1-background, design considerations, and model development. Ann Thorac Surg 2018;105(5):1411–8.

25. Moonesinghe SR, Bashford T, Wagstaff D. Implementing risk calculators: time for the Trojan Horse? Br J Anaesth 2018;121(6):1192–6.

26. Liu Y, Cohen ME, Hall BL, et al. Evaluation and enhancement of calibration in the American College of Surgeons NSQIP Surgical Risk Calculator. J Am Coll Surg 2016;223(2):231–9.

27. Sacks GD, Dawes AJ, Ettner SL, et al. Impact of a risk calculator on risk perception and surgical decision making: a randomized trial. Ann Surg 2016;264(6): 889–95.
28. Leeds IL, Rosenblum AJ, Wise PE, et al. Eye of the beholder: risk calculators and barriers to adoption in surgical trainees. Surgery 2018;164(5):1117–23.
29. Krittanawong C, Zhang H, Wang Z, et al. Artificial intelligence in precision cardiovascular medicine. J Am Coll Cardiol 2017;69(21):2657–64.
30. Cook NR, Ridker PM. Calibration of the pooled cohort equations for atherosclerotic cardiovascular disease: an update. Ann Intern Med 2016;165(11):786–94.
31. Bishop CM. Pattern recognition and machine learning (information science and statistics). New York: Springer-Verlag; 2006.
32. Ciompi F, Chung K, van Riel SJ, et al. Towards automatic pulmonary nodule management in lung cancer screening with deep learning. Sci Rep 2017;7:46479.
33. Lip GY, Nieuwlaat R, Pisters R, et al. Refining clinical risk stratification for predicting stroke and thromboembolism in atrial fibrillation using a novel risk factor-based approach: the Euro Heart Survey on Atrial Fibrillation. Chest 2010; 137(2):263–72.
34. Deo RC. Machine learning in medicine. Circulation 2015;132(20):1920–30.
35. Lo-Ciganic WH, Huang JL, Zhang HH, et al. Evaluation of machine-learning algorithms for predicting opioid overdose risk among Medicare beneficiaries with opioid prescriptions. JAMA Netw Open 2019;2(3):e190968.
36. Hsich E, Gorodeski EZ, Blackstone EH, et al. Identifying important risk factors for survival in patient with systolic heart failure using random survival forests. Circ Cardiovasc Qual Outcomes 2011;4(1):39–45.
37. Chirikov VV, Shaya FT, Onukwugha E, et al. Tree-based claims algorithm for measuring pretreatment quality of care in Medicare disabled hepatitis C patients. Med Care 2017;55(12):e104–12.
38. Thottakkara P, Ozrazgat-Baslanti T, Hupf BB, et al. Application of machine learning techniques to high-dimensional clinical data to forecast postoperative complications. PLoS One 2016;11(5):e0155705.
39. Karadaghy OA, Shew M, New J, et al. Development and assessment of a machine learning model to help predict survival among patients with oral squamous cell carcinoma. JAMA Otolaryngol Head Neck Surg 2019;145(12):1115–20.
40. Bihorac A, Ozrazgat-Baslanti T, Ebadi A, et al. MySurgeryRisk: development and validation of a machine-learning risk algorithm for major complications and death after surgery. Ann Surg 2019;269(4):652–62.
41. Bertsimas D, Dunn J, Velmahos GC, et al. Surgical risk is not linear: derivation and validation of a novel, user-friendly, and machine-learning-based predictive OpTimal Trees in Emergency Surgery Risk (POTTER) Calculator. Ann Surg 2018;268(4):574–83.

Safety of Surgical Telehealth in the Outpatient and Inpatient Setting

Shawn Purnell, MD, MS, Feibi Zheng, MD, MBA*

KEYWORDS

- Telehealth • Telemedicine • mHealth • Surgical safety

KEY POINTS

- Telemedicine replacement for routine in-person postoperative care appears to be safe for carefully selected low-risk patients undergoing low-risk procedures.
- High-quality trials studying telehealth interventions to improve patient safety and patient outcomes are ongoing in all surgical subspecialties.
- Telehealth interventions must be designed in an iterative fashion with consideration for local resources, processes, and end-user patient preferences and needs.

INTRODUCTION

The COVID-19 pandemic has accelerated the adoption of telehealth in all phases of surgical care (**Table 1**). Both CMS and commercial payers have loosened guidelines for billing and reimbursement in both the inpatient and the outpatient settings. Medicare has waived originating site requirements, which previously required reimbursed care to be provided to patients in health care shortage or rural areas and for the visits to be conducted with the patient physically present at a remote health care facility. Before the COVID-19 crisis, telemedicine could not be provided across state lines unless the surgeon had a license to practice in the neighboring state. Since April 2020, state licensing requirements have been loosened in order to provide increased flexibility to provide care across state lines. Most states have also implemented telemedicine parity laws, which allow for synchronous video visits to be reimbursed at the same rate as in-person visits for both established and new patient visits. These rapid developments necessitate an examination of the safety of telehealth platforms and interventions that are proliferating globally.

Department of Surgery, Houston Methodist Hospital, 6550 Fannin Street, Smith 16, Houston, TX 77030, USA
* Corresponding author.
E-mail address: fzheng@houstonmethodist.org

Surg Clin N Am 101 (2021) 109–119
https://doi.org/10.1016/j.suc.2020.09.003
0039-6109/21/© 2020 Elsevier Inc. All rights reserved.

Table 1 Key definitions	
Telehealth	Digital health care activities, platforms, services
Telemedicine	Remote diagnosis and treatment of patients by means of telecommunication technology
mHealth	Use of smartphones and tablets for telehealth
Remote patient monitoring	The use of wearable devices, mobile devices, applications for physiologic data transmission, analysis, and monitoring
Tele-ICU	A platform that uses remote patient monitoring technology to augment care of intensive care unit patients

Data from NEJM Catalyst. What is Telehealth? *Massachusetts Medical Society.* 2018. Available at: https://catalyst.nejm.org/doi/full/10.1056/CAT.18.0268.

EVALUATION OF TELEHEALTH FOR PATIENT SAFETY

There is no widely accepted framework for the evaluation of telehealth interventions or platforms. However, most frameworks examine the following outcomes: patient access and acceptability, surgeon and staff satisfaction, efficacy of intervention, safety of intervention, patient-reported outcomes and use of institutional resources to deploy intervention, and cost-effectiveness. Additional domains related to the development of the intervention include stakeholder input, interoperability with existing electronic medical record (EMR) software, and data security and governance.[1]

TELEHEALTH IN THE OUTPATIENT SETTING

Telehealth modalities in the outpatient setting, which have been previously studied, include substitution of in-person visits for routine postoperative care, patient education, medication adherence, and home-based virtual ward recovery programs. Many of these programs have been evaluated for feasibility and safety in carefully selected populations. The authors examine several of these programs across different surgical subspecialties in later discussion.

The Veterans Administration was an early adopter of telemedicine technologies. It was one of the first hospital systems to evaluate the safety of telemedicine for routine postoperative care for low-risk procedures.[2] Eisenberg and colleagues[3] examined 62 patients undergoing laparoscopic inguinal hernia repair. These patients were given a telephone-only postoperative visit. Eighty-nine percent of patients were able to successfully complete the visit; 5% never completed any follow-up visit, and 7% were accidentally scheduled an in-person visit. Of the patients who had a telephone-only postoperative visit, 9% returned for an in-person visit for issues that could not be addressed via the telephone visit. One was found to have an early recurrence, and one was found to have a seroma.

More recently, in a randomized prospective trial, a tertiary care hospital in Spain randomized 200 carefully selected patients to telemedicine follow-up video visits or in-person office follow-up visits. The 3 most commonly performed procedures in this group of patients were laparoscopic cholecystectomy, inguinal hernia repair, and laparoscopic appendectomy. In their primary endpoint of successful completion of the assigned visit type, 90% of the patients in the in-person visit and 74% of patients in the virtual visit arm were able to complete their assigned visit type. There were no differences in the secondary outcomes or need for additional clinic or emergency department (ED) visits or patient satisfaction.[4] In another randomized Canadian trial of 65 women undergoing breast reconstruction, the intervention group was assigned to receive postoperative care via mobile app versus usual standard of care, which consisted of in-person postoperative visits at week 1 and week 4. Through the app, the patients were instructed to submit photographs of the surgical site, respond to an analog visual pain scale, and fill out a quality of recovery survey with daily asynchronous monitoring for the first 2 weeks and then weekly monitoring for the subsequent 2 weeks. The mobile app group reported a decreased need for in-person visits and no difference in rates of postoperative complications, which were surgical site infection and seroma.[5]

In a virtual care home recovery study, 30 patients were randomized after minimally invasive colectomy to standard of care enhanced recovery after surgery (ERAS) protocol or ERAS protocol with preplanned accelerated discharge on postoperative day 1 with home recovery monitoring using a tablet computer with a planned postoperative video televisit on postoperative day 2 and instant messaging with the care team as needed. Most of the patients in the accelerated discharge arm were able to safely recover at home, with 4 patients returning to the ED for abdominal pain, *Clostridium difficile* colitis, anastomotic leak, and port site hernia. None of these complications were attributed to accelerated discharge, and use of the app did not result in a delay in needed care.[6]

Further examples of randomized clinical trials involving telemedicine interventions in various surgical specialties are highlighted in **Table 2**.

PATIENT SAFETY OPPORTUNITIES IN THE OUTPATIENT SETTING

These studies demonstrate that in carefully selected patients, telemedicine interventions to replace and augment routine postoperative care are safe, are feasible, and may improve patient satisfaction when compared with routine in-person postoperative care. The low risk of complications in these studies also calls into question whether routine follow-up with a surgeon is necessary in most low-risk patients undergoing low-risk surgery. Very few studies show the ability of these interventions to enhance clinical outcomes or decrease complications. Lee and colleagues'[10] study was one of the few studies that demonstrated an improvement in 90-day readmissions in a liver transplant population using a tablet computer coupled with vital sign monitoring and on-demand instant messaging, phone calls, and video encounters with the care team (28% vs 58%; $P = .004$). The value of telemedicine interventions in improving patient safety may be better demonstrated in higher-risk surgeries and higher-risk populations where there is greater variance in outcomes.

Many telehealth interventions for the postoperative phase of care were initially focused on substitution of care for follow-up. However, as pressure for value-based payment grows, more recent studies have focused on new telehealth strategies to improve length of stay while maintaining or improving patient safety during the recovery phase and preventing readmissions. Although telehealth interventions have demonstrated potential savings to patients in terms of time and travel costs in the outpatient setting, few studies have examined the return on investment from the institutional or surgeon perspective. The few economic studies of telemedicine in postoperative care have focused on reallocation of provider time or improved clinic access.[17,18]

Another area of potential study is whether telehealth platforms can predict impending complications. In a prospective cohort study, Panda and colleagues[19] captured smartphone accelerometer data from 1 week before surgery to 6 months after surgery in patients with cancer. Accelerometer data were used as a proxy measure of physical

Table 2
Randomized controlled trials in the evaluation of telemedicine applications in the outpatient setting

Surgical Discipline	Procedure Types	Intervention	Outcomes	References
General surgery	Inguinal hernia, laparoscopic cholecystectomy, laparoscopic appendectomy	Video follow-up visit vs in-person visit	Feasibility of completing scheduled visit type. No difference in 30-d complications, 30-d ED visits, or patient satisfaction	Cremades et al,[4] 2020
	Stoma creation	Stoma nurse follow-up by teleconsultation video visit with patient presenting to district medical center vs in-person visit at university hospital	No differences in quality of life as measured by EQ-5D index, number of 30-d hospital appointments or readmissions; communication rated as poorer in the teleconsultation group	Augestad et al,[7] 2020
Surgical oncology	Colectomy	Accelerated discharge after ERAS protocol with computer tablet remote monitoring vs standard ERAS protocol	Lower length of stay in accelerated discharge group without increase in severe adverse events	Bednarski et al,[6] 2019
Plastic surgery	Breast reconstruction	Smartphone app with 1-way pain reporting and incision photograph submission in lieu of in-person visit	No difference in 30-d in-person visits composite (PCP, ED, surgeon), 30-d complications, or patient satisfaction scores	Armstrong et al,[5] 2017
Thoracic surgery	Thoracotomy	Automated telephone calls to the patient for symptom monitoring with e-mail alert to care team for severity triggers vs monitoring without e-mail to clinicians	Reduction in number of reports of severe symptoms	Cleeland et al,[8] 2011
Transplant surgery	Kidney transplant	Smartphone app integrated with wireless blood pressure monitor and medication box	Improved medication adherence and systolic blood pressure measurement at months 1 and 3	McGillicuddy et al,[9] 2013

Specialty	Procedure	Intervention	Outcomes	Study
	Liver transplant	Tablet computer with vital sign transmission, on demand instant messaging and video visit vs standard of care	Lower 90-d readmission rate	Lee et al,[10] 2019
Urology	Prostatectomy	Video visit in lieu of in-person visit	Equivalent visit efficiency, patient satisfaction; decreased patient cost	Viers et al,[11] 2015
Orthopedic surgery	Rotator cuff repair	Video visit in lieu of in-person visit	Detection of surgical site drainage in 3 patients in telehealth group, 4 in control group; 1 patient in telemedicine group with postoperative myocardial infarction; similar pain scores and patient satisfaction	Kane et al,[12] 2020
	Total knee replacement	Smartphone app with daily instruction via push notification vs smartphone app with twice a week instruction (information provided across 2 groups are the same)	Lower pain scores, higher quality of life, activities of daily living, and patient satisfaction in the daily instruction group	Timmers et al,[13] 2019
Vascular	Lower-extremity revascularization via groin incision	Telehealth electronic monitoring system including tablet computer for image capture, weight scale, blood pressure cuff, thermometer, and pulse oximeter reviewed by care manager vs usual standard of care with no remote monitoring	No difference in 30-d readmissions or surgical site infection; increased patient satisfaction in intervention group	Mousa et al,[14] 2019
Gynecology	Pelvic floor surgery	Telephone interviews vs in-person visit for postoperative care	No difference in adverse events, ED visits, or PCP visits	Thompson et al,[15] 2019
Pediatric surgery	Nonoperative and operative hospitalization	Video visit vs in-person follow-up	No missed clinical findings in video visit group; travel time, days off from school/work lower in the telemedicine group	Goedeke et al,[16] 2019

Data from Refs.[4–16]

activity. Twenty-seven percent of patients had at least 1 postoperative event, which included readmission, ED visit, wound complication, reoperation, respiratory complication, sepsis, and death. Before surgery, physical activity levels as measured through accelerometer data were similar between groups with and without postoperative events. However, postoperative accelerometer data demonstrated a decreased level of activity in the group with a postoperative event.

Although telemedicine has been used on a limited basis for preoperative triage, no randomized trials have been performed to date to evaluate the safety of telemedicine consultation in the preoperative setting. Before the COVID-19 pandemic, many US states prohibited the use of telemedicine for initial consultation. Since then, state regulations have rapidly evolved to accommodate new patient visits. Studies carried out over the next 2 years will likely determine which patients and procedures can be safely brought to the operating room without an in-person physical examination at the time of initial consultation.

FUTURE DIRECTIONS IN OUTPATIENT TELEHEALTH

Although 80% of Americans use smartphones or tablets, it is important to recognize that new technologies may exacerbate existing disparities.[20] Initial pilots of new programs may only be designed for English speakers and rely on patients to have access to self-purchased home-monitoring equipment or mHealth devices. This need may disadvantage minority, immigrant, nontechnologically adept, and low-income patients.[5,21] Furthermore, results from such trials may not be generalizable to wider populations and may fail to show safety equivalence or improved outcomes when more broadly implemented.

Design of future telemedicine interventions must take into account patient preferences and limitations. For example, the effect of smartphone applications on medication compliance after transplant surgery has been studied in multiple studies with varying results.[22,23] Some studies report low levels of engagement with the application limiting the effectiveness of potential interventions, whereas others show sustained improvements not only in medication adherence but also in clinical outcomes. In Timmers and colleagues,[13] the same patient volume and content of educational material were given to total knee replacement patients in both arms of the study through a smartphone application with the only difference being the format and frequency of instruction. This study suggests that the timing, volume, and delivery format of the information make a difference in patient-reported outcomes.

TELE-INTENSIVE CARE UNITS

Intensive care units (ICUs) across the country are under substantial strain because of the relative shortage of intensivist physicians and increasing US elderly population requiring complex levels of care.[24] Most ICUs in the United States are unable to be staffed by intensivists, despite evidence from multiple studies that intensivist-staffed ICUs have both lower length of stays and mortalities.[25,26] In addition to the shortage of intensivists, burnout plays a significant role in intensivist productivity and longevity. Guntupalli and Fromm[27] studied emotional exhaustion, depersonalization, and personal accomplishment using the Maslach Burnout Inventory, in which one-third of intensivists scored in the high range. In order to "battle intensivist burnout," research has focused on workload management through tele-ICU implementation and improved workflows rather than merely relying on resilience training.[28]

Tele-ICUs leverage an intensivist's care across multiple ICUs, significantly decreasing workload. A remote intensivist is able to care for distant patients in multiple

ICUs via an audiovisual interface, document findings within an EMR, and administer treatments via computerized physician order entry tools. Initial technology used tele-conferencing video and spacelabs bedside data to provide remote intensivist access to patients.[29] Today, advances in technology continue to expand tele-ICU technologies while driving down costs, making tele-ICU more scalable. In addition, tele-ICU can be categorized into continuous, episodic, and response care models that are tailored to the hospitals' needs.[30] Although technology plays an integral role in tele-ICU, successful implementation is also contingent on patient and staff acceptance, as well as organizational management.

Tele-ICU uses audio-video technology, telemetry, and EMRs to allow a centralized intensivist to care for multiple distant ICUs.[31] Early attempts at tele-ICU were curtailed by a lack of technology and high costs. Rosenfeld and colleagues[29] were one of the first groups to trial tele-ICU on a large scale in 1997, evaluating the feasibility of 24-hour telemedicine coverage in a 10-bed surgical ICU. They performed an observational time series triple cohort study over 16 weeks and found that 24-hour telemedicine coverage decreased length of stay, costs, complications, and mortality. The Rosenfeld and colleagues study served as a proof-of-concept model, confirming that tele-ICU is feasible and improves overall quality of care for the patients.

Lilly and colleagues[32] performed a single-academic center prospective study of 6290 adults across 7 ICUs comparing preintervention traditional ICUs and postintervention tele-ICUs. The postintervention tele-ICUs were associated with increased adherence to best practice guidelines, lower rates of preventable complications, shorter lengths of stay, and decreased mortality. However, a multi-institutional observational pre-post study by Nassar and colleagues[33] in 2012 found no significant decreases in mortality or length of stay. Nassar and colleagues and Lilly and colleagues highlight the complexity of tele-ICU implementation across complex health care systems. Tele-ICU implementation requires reengineering of the ICU to integrate technology, standards of care, and cultural change within individual health care organizations.

Three metaanalyses have been performed on tele-ICU interventions examining mortality and length of stay. In 2011, Young and colleagues[34] identified 13 studies from 35 ICUs revealing a decrease in ICU and hospital mortality, and ICU length of stay. Hospital length of stay was not significantly decreased following tele-ICU intervention. Chen and colleagues[35] revealed similar results in 2018, showing a reduction in ICU mortality, hospital mortality, and ICU length of stay, but no significant reduction in hospital length of stay (confidence interval −1.14 to −0.59 days) following tele-ICU implementation. Wilcox and Adhikari[36] included 11 observational studies showing tele-ICU was associated with lower overall hospital and ICU mortalities, and lower ICU lengths of stay. However, these results must be taken with caution, as nonrandomized trials can overestimate significant results. Hospitals must also be careful to tailor tele-ICUs technology and workflow to their organization, as there is no one-size-fits-all tele-ICU model.

PATIENT SAFETY OPPORTUNITIES IN TELE-INTENSIVE CARE UNITS

The recent advent of tele-ICU has led to the development of a unique set of patient safety advancements and concerns. Outside of mortality and length of stay outcomes, tele-ICU has improved patient safety through adherence to standard of care. Pre-post tele-ICU interventional studies have shown improved adherence for deep vein thrombosis prophylaxis (odds ratio [OR] 15.4), stress ulcer prophylaxis (OR 4.57), cardiovascular protection (OR 30.7), and ventilator-associated pneumonia (OR 2.2).[32] The overall tele-ICU decrease in patient mortality and length may be attributed to both the adherence to standard of care best practices and the tele-ICU technologies.

In addition, tele-ICU can improve patient care through the use of team-based systems. Patient monitoring technology has significantly increased ICU staff alerts with a single 10-bed ICU study showing as many as 100,000 alarms per year. Tele-ICU systems can include centralized command centers staffed with nurses and physicians who are able to better monitor and readily respond to critical patient alerts. Traditional ICUs respond to a threshold 90% of critical alarms within 3 minutes 45% of the time, compared with tele-ICUs that respond to 71% (P<.001).[37] Importantly, studies show that ICUs with response times less than 3 minutes have shorter lengths of stay for ICU patients.[38] Comparing traditional ICU care with supplemental tele-ICU, studies show a noninferiority or improved patient care in favor of supplemental tele-ICU care.

Tele-ICU medicine moves away from the traditional doctor-patient relationship, and research regarding its effect on patient satisfaction is lacking. Patient and family satisfaction has been shown to be dependent on the understanding that both care teams, on-site and remote, are present to care for the patient.[39] No standardized tools have been developed to properly assess satisfaction in the tele-ICU (**Box 1**).

FUTURE DIRECTIONS IN TELE-INTENSIVE CARE UNITS

Future tele-ICU studies are focused on technology integration, data analysis, and systems implementation. Current tele-ICU technology relies on multiple platforms to integrate patient information regarding radiology, documentation, and order entry.[40] Integration will help standardize best practices and nomenclature across institutions, allowing for improved analysis of tele-ICU effectiveness.

The COVID-19 pandemic has also created an opportunity to study not only patient safety but also health care worker safety in the context of tele-ICU. Tele-ICU may minimize some of the need for physical interaction between the patient and the caregiver, save personal protective equipment, and prevent the spread of nosocomial infection between patients. Tele-ICU can also enable family members to visit with ventilated, isolated patients without exposing the bedside nurse. Furthermore, tele-ICU can be used to reallocate intensivists to areas of greater need during surge events.

Intensivists have the daunting task of analyzing vast amounts of patient information produced by tele-ICU technologies on multiple platforms to help guide patient care. Machine learning (ML) software is being developed to help establish connections between the vast heterogenous information to guide patient care. Current ML software uses classical models that can detect sepsis early, identify light versus deep sedation in mechanically ventilated patients, and predict the risk of hospital-acquired pressure ulcers.[41] Newer ML models use deep neural networks centered on novel algorithms that better integrate large and heterogenous data.[42]

Last, with improvements in technology integration and data analysis must come system implementation strategies. Differences between mortality and length of stay in Lilly and colleagues[32] and Nassar and colleagues[33] emphasize that tele-ICU

Box 1
General applications of tele-intensive care units

Extension of limited local workforce

Remote consultation/supervision

Family visits in patients under isolation precautions (such as COVID-19)

success depends on proper implementation. Implementation requires successful change in behavior, acceptance from all staff, and an extensive information support system. Future studies are needed on managerial organization, clearly defined tele-ICU implementation steps, and examination of individual steps that are improving patient care.[42]

SUMMARY

Pilot studies and small clinical trials have demonstrated the feasibility and safety of telehealth interventions in both the inpatient and the outpatient setting. The next iteration of outpatient telehealth evaluation should focus on expanding telehealth studies to more diverse populations, evaluating the cost-effectiveness of these interventions, and seeking to demonstrate improved outcomes rather than equivalence. For inpatient telehealth, tele-ICU shows promise to improve adherence to best practices and enables better outcomes by sorting and prioritizing information for intensivists. Future design of telehealth interventions must also address interoperability standards, user preferences and needs, and data privacy and ownership issues.

CLINICS CARE POINTS

- Telemedicine visits may be safe in lieu of in-person visits for low-risk surgeries in low-risk patients and is well accepted by patients.
- Tele-ICUs may improve efficiency of allocation of scarce intensivist resources and shows promise to improve adherence to evidence-based practices.
- Design of telehealth platforms in the inpatient and outpatient setting must take into account institutional resources and culture, staff acceptance and training, user interface, and adult learning principles.

DISCLOSURE

The authors have nothing to disclose.

REFERENCES

1. Hebert M. Telehealth success: evaluation framework development. Stud Health Technol Inform 2001;84(Pt 2):1145–9.
2. Hwa K, Wren SM. Telehealth follow-up in lieu of postoperative clinic visit for ambulatory surgery: results of a pilot program. JAMA Surg 2013;148(9):823–7.
3. Eisenberg D, Hwa K, Wren SM. Telephone follow-up by a midlevel provider after laparoscopic inguinal hernia repair instead of face-to-face clinic visit. JSLS 2015; 19(1). e2014.00205.
4. Cremades M, Ferret G, Pares D, et al. Telemedicine to follow patients in a general surgery department. A randomized controlled trial. Am J Surg 2020;219(6): 882–7.
5. Armstrong KA, Coyte PC, Brown M, et al. Effect of home monitoring via mobile app on the number of in-person visits following ambulatory surgery: a randomized clinical trial. JAMA Surg 2017;152(7):622–7.
6. Bednarski BK, Nickerson TP, You YN, et al. Randomized clinical trial of accelerated enhanced recovery after minimally invasive colorectal cancer surgery (RecoverMI trial). Br J Surg 2019;106(10):1311–8.
7. Augestad KM, Sneve AM, Lindsetmo RO. Telemedicine in postoperative follow-up of STOMa PAtients: a randomized clinical trial (the STOMPA trial). Br J Surg 2020;107(5):509–18.

8. Cleeland CS, Wang XS, Shi Q, et al. Automated symptom alerts reduce postoperative symptom severity after cancer surgery: a randomized controlled clinical trial. J Clin Oncol 2011;29(8):994–1000.

9. McGillicuddy JW, Gregoski MJ, Weiland AK, et al. Mobile health medication adherence and blood pressure control in renal transplant recipients: a proof-of-concept randomized controlled trial. JMIR Res Protoc 2013;2(2):e32.

10. Lee TC, Kaiser TE, Alloway R, et al. Telemedicine based remote home monitoring after liver transplantation: results of a randomized prospective trial. Ann Surg 2019;270(3):564–72.

11. Viers BR, Lightner DJ, Rivera ME, et al. Efficiency, satisfaction, and costs for remote video visits following radical prostatectomy: a randomized controlled trial. Eur Urol 2015;68(4):729–35.

12. Kane LT, Thakar O, Jamgochian G, et al. The role of telehealth as a platform for postoperative visits following rotator cuff repair: a prospective, randomized controlled trial. J Shoulder Elbow Surg 2020;29(4):775–83.

13. Timmers T, Janssen L, van der Weegen W, et al. The effect of an app for day-to-day postoperative care education on patients with total knee replacement: randomized controlled trial. JMIR MHealth UHealth 2019;7(10):e15323.

14. Mousa AY, Broce M, Monnett S, et al. Results of telehealth electronic monitoring for post discharge complications and surgical site infections following arterial revascularization with groin incision. Ann Vasc Surg 2019;57:160–9.

15. Thompson JC, Cichowski SB, Rogers RG, et al. Outpatient visits versus telephone interviews for postoperative care: a randomized controlled trial. Int Urogynecol J 2019;30(10):1639–46.

16. Goedeke J, Ertl A, Zoller D, et al. Telemedicine for pediatric surgical outpatient follow-up: a prospective, randomized single-center trial. J Pediatr Surg 2019; 54(1):200–7.

17. Zheng F, Park KW, Thi WJ, et al. Financial implications of telemedicine visits in an academic endocrine surgery program. Surgery 2019;165(3):617–21.

18. Nikolian VC, Williams AM, Jacobs BN, et al. Pilot study to evaluate the safety, feasibility, and financial implications of a postoperative telemedicine program. Ann Surg 2018;268(4):700–7.

19. Panda N, Solsky I, Huang EJ, et al. Using smartphones to capture novel recovery metrics after cancer surgery. JAMA Surg 2019;155(2):123–9.

20. Smartphones in the U.S. - Statistics & Facts. Available at: https://nam03.safelinks. protection.outlook.com/.

21. Gunter RL, Chouinard S, Fernandes-Taylor S, et al. Current use of telemedicine for post-discharge surgical care: a systematic review. J Am Coll Surg 2016; 222(5):915–27.

22. Gomis-Pastor M, Roig E, Mirabet S, et al. A mobile app (mHeart) to detect medication nonadherence in the heart transplant population: validation study. JMIR MHealth UHealth 2020;8(2):e15957.

23. Han A, Min SI, Ahn S, et al. Mobile medication manager application to improve adherence with immunosuppressive therapy in renal transplant recipients: a randomized controlled trial. PLoS One 2019;14(11):e0224595.

24. Lois M. The shortage of critical care physicians: is there a solution? J Crit Care 2014;29(6):1121–2.

25. Angus DC, Kelley MA, Schmitz RJ, et al, Committee on manpower for pulmonary and critical care societies (COMPACCS). Caring for the critically ill patient. Current and projected workforce requirements for care of the critically ill and patients

with pulmonary disease: can we meet the requirements of an aging population? JAMA 2000;284(21):2762–70.

26. Pronovost PJ, Angus DC, Dorman T, et al. Physician staffing patterns and clinical outcomes in critically ill patients: a systematic review. JAMA 2002;288(17): 2151–62.

27. Guntupalli KK, Fromm RE. Burnout in the internist–intensivist. Intensive Care Med 1996;22(7):625–30.

28. Lilly CM, Cucchi E, Marshall N, et al. Battling intensivist burnout: a role for workload management. Chest 2019;156(5):1001–7.

29. Rosenfeld BA, Dorman T, Breslow MJ, et al. Intensive care unit telemedicine: alternate paradigm for providing continuous intensivist care. Crit Care Med 2000;28(12):3925–31.

30. Herasevich V, Subramanian S. Tele-ICU technologies. Crit Care Clin 2019;35(3): 427–38.

31. Kumar G, Falk DM, Bonello RS, et al. The costs of critical care telemedicine programs: a systematic review and analysis. Chest 2013;143(1):19–29.

32. Lilly CM, Cody S, Zhao H, et al. Hospital mortality, length of stay, and preventable complications among critically ill patients before and after tele-ICU reengineering of critical care processes. JAMA 2011;305(21):2175–83.

33. Nassar BS, Vaughan-Sarrazin MS, Jiang L, et al. Impact of an intensive care unit telemedicine program on patient outcomes in an integrated health care system. JAMA Intern Med 2014;174(7):1160–7.

34. Young LB, Chan PS, Lu X, et al. Impact of telemedicine intensive care unit coverage on patient outcomes: a systematic review and meta-analysis. Arch Intern Med 2011;171(6):498–506.

35. Chen J, Sun D, Yang W, et al. Clinical and economic outcomes of telemedicine programs in the intensive care unit: a systematic review and meta-analysis. J Intensive Care Med 2018;33(7):383–93.

36. Wilcox ME, Adhikari NKJ. The effect of telemedicine in critically ill patients: systematic review and meta-analysis. Crit Care 2012;16(4):R127.

37. Lilly CM, Fisher KA, Ries M, et al. A national ICU telemedicine survey: validation and results. Chest 2012;142(1):40–7.

38. Fuhrman SA, Lilly CM. ICU telemedicine solutions. Clin Chest Med 2015;36(3): 401–7.

39. Golembeski S, Willmitch B, Kim SS. Perceptions of the care experience in critical care units enhanced by a tele-ICU. AACN Adv Crit Care 2012;23(3):323–9.

40. Sapirstein A, Lone N, Latif A, et al. Tele ICU: paradox or panacea? Best Pract Res Clin Anaesthesiol 2009;23(1):115–26.

41. Kindle RD, Badawi O, Celi LA, et al. Intensive care unit telemedicine in the era of big data, artificial intelligence, and computer clinical decision support systems. Crit Care Clin 2019;35(3):483–95.

42. Lilly CM, Zubrow MT, Kempner KM, et al. Critical care telemedicine: evolution and state of the art. Crit Care Med 2014;42(11):2429–36.

Administrative and Registry Databases for Patient Safety Tracking and Quality Improvement

Brian C. Brajcich, MD, MS[a,b,1], Chelsea P. Fischer, MD, MS[a,c,*,1],
Clifford Y. Ko, MD, MS, MSHS, FSCRS[a,d]

KEYWORDS

- Quality improvement • Datasets • Quality infrastructure • Patient safety

KEY POINTS

- Datasets are an essential tool for monitoring patient safety and complications and can also be used to drive quality improvement.
- Multiple types of datasets are available, each with its strengths and weaknesses.
- Data alone are insufficient for meaningful quality improvement. Infrastructure is essential to ensure action from data.
- Rapid technological advancement, such as machine learning, and profound increase in data quantity necessitate flexibility and continuous learning on the part of quality improvement practitioners.

INTRODUCTION

Outcome measurement has an extensive history in the surgical profession, dating back more than 100 years to Ernest Codman recording and publishing outcomes for patients—his so called "End Results Idea."[1,2] He went as far as to found his own hospital—the End Results Hospital—and published the outcomes of all of the patients treated there, including errors in diagnosis or treatment.[3] Although his efforts to enact widespread quality measurement and reporting were not widely accepted at the time, the principles he championed have persisted and revolutionized surgical care today.

Funding: BCB and CPF are supported by the American College of Surgeons as part of the Clinical Scholars in Residence Program. CYK receives salary support from the American College of Surgeons.
[a] Division of Research and Optimal Patient Care, American College of Surgeons, 633 North St. Clair Street, 23Road Floor, Chicago, IL 60611, USA; [b] Department of Surgery, Surgical Outcomes and Quality Improvement Center (SOQIC), Northwestern Medicine, Chicago, IL, USA; [c] Loyola University Medical Center, Maywood, IL, USA; [d] UCLA Medical Center, Los Angeles, CA, USA
[1] BCB and CPF acted as co-first authors on this publication.
* Corresponding author:
E-mail address: cfischer@facs.org

Surg Clin N Am 101 (2021) 121–134
https://doi.org/10.1016/j.suc.2020.09.010
surgical.theclinics.com

In addition to being credited with inspiring modern morbidity and mortality conferences, the current emphasis on quality and outcomes in surgical care is attributable to his work. Today, surgical outcomes are measured for hospital accreditation processes, epidemiologic monitoring of disease, reimbursement, and creation of hospital ratings. As a byproduct of these activities, a large quantity of surgical outcome data is generated and stored in datasets. Increasingly, these datasets are being used not only to measure outcomes but to drive and monitor surgical quality improvement (QI).

TYPES OF SURGICAL DATASETS

Datasets used for measurement of surgical outcomes may be categorized into 3 major groups. First are administrative datasets, which are usually generated from claims data submitted for billing purposes and contain information about diagnoses and treatments. Second are clinical registries, which contain clinical information abstracted from medical records, usually by a trained clinical abstractor. Finally, local datasets are usually prospectively collected and often specific to a disease or procedure type. Because this third type of dataset tends to be individualized to the local setting, it will not be explored in detail in this article.

A common function of administrative data is to facilitate submission of billing claims to various payers. Medical encounter records are assigned International Classification of Diseases (ICD) or Current Procedural Terminology (CPT) codes and contain extensive information on procedures, diagnosis, and resource utilization. Collection of data across multiple encounters allows longitudinal tracking of patient outcomes in some administrative datasets. With clinical outcomes increasingly used to determine reimbursement, they are now a focus of administrative databases as well. Examples of national administrative datasets include the National Inpatient Sample developed as part of the Agency for Healthcare Research and Quality Healthcare Cost and Utilization Project, the Centers for Medicare & Medicaid Services (CMS) databases, and private claims databases such as Vizient or Premier. There are limits to the generalizability of these databases; for example, CMS only contains information about patients who are Medicare or Medicaid recipients.[4] Private databases include both public and private insurance billing information with automated abstraction from electronic medical records. The private databases have many subscribers and provide the ability to benchmark performance.[5,6] Although these databases' primary purpose is to track resource utilization, some can also be used for QI without incurring additional institutional costs.

In contrast to administrative databases, clinical registries exist primarily to capture clinical care in more detail than can be recorded simply by ICD and CPT codes. The purpose of these data may include monitoring disease epidemiology or practice patterns, measuring adherence to specific quality measures, or guiding and monitoring QI efforts. Data are abstracted at each contributing site by clinical registrars who are often trained in proper identification and coding of patient characteristics, diagnoses, procedures, and outcomes.[7] Because of this process, clinical registries can focus more specifically on clinical areas, such as cardiac surgery, bariatric surgery, trauma, cancer, or short-term postoperative outcomes. Some clinical registry abstractors will contact patients directly or review governmental death records to obtain follow-up information that is not captured in the medical record.[7] **Table 1** provides a partial list of currently available registries with surgical data.

CLINICAL REGISTRIES

The underlying principle of a clinical registry reflects the idea of Ernest Codman that a system can track adverse outcomes and identify the underlying problems or practices

Table 1 US surgical clinical registries	
Surgical Specialty	**Clinical Registries**
General Surgery	ACS NSQIP Washington State's Surgical Care and Outcomes Assessment Program American Hernia Society
Surgical Oncology	National Cancer Database NCCN Oncology Outcomes Database
Trauma Surgery	North Carolina State Trauma Registry National Trauma Data Bank
Endocrine Surgery	Collaborative Endocrine Surgery Quality Improvement Program (CESQIP)
Burn Surgery	American Burn Association Registry
Abdominal Transplant Surgery	UNOS Scientific Registry Transplant Recipient Scientific Registry of Transplant Recipients
Vascular Surgery	Society for Vascular Surgery Vascular Registry Society for Vascular Surgery Vascular Quality Initiative Registry
Bariatric Surgery	Metabolic and Bariatric Surgery Accreditation and Quality Improvement Program Bariatric Outcomes Longitudinal Database Michigan Bariatric Surgery Collaborative
Pediatric Surgery	Pediatric NSQIP
Orthopedic Surgery	Function and Outcomes Research for Comparative Effectiveness in Total Joint Replacement (FORCE TJR) American Joint Replacement Registry (AJRR) North American Spine Society (NASS) Registry
Urology	Michigan Urological Surgery Improvement Collaborative (MUSIC) Cancer of the Prostate Strategic Urologic Research Endeavor (CaPSURE) American Urological Association Registry (AQUA) Program
Neurologic Surgery	National Neurosurgery Quality and Outcomes Database (N2QOD) North American Spine Society (NASS) Registry
Cardiothoracic Surgery	VA Continuous Improvement in Cardiac Surgery Program Northern New England Cardiovascular Study Group Society of Thoracic Surgeons National Adult Cardiac Database New York State Coronary Artery Bypass Registry Society of Thoracic Surgeons General Thoracic surgery Database
Otolaryngology	American Academy of Otolaryngology Reg-ent Clinical Data Registry
Ophthalmology	American Academy of Ophthalmology IRIS Registry
Gynecologic Surgery	Society of Gynecologic Oncology Clinical Outcomes Registry
Plastic Surgery	American Society of Plastic Surgeons Tracking Operations and Outcomes for Plastic Surgeons (TOPS)

Abbreviations: ACS, American College of Surgeons; NA, not available; NCCN, National Comprehensive Cancer Network; UNOS, United Network for Organ Sharing; VA, veterans affairs.

that cause them. Clinical registries are often specific to a disease process or patient populations (see **Table 1**). Some of the most commonly used registries in QI are described in detail here.

The National Cancer Database (NCDB), an effort by the American College of Surgeons (ACS) Commission on Cancer (CoC), was founded in 1989 to track trends in cancer care, provide data to create and monitor adherence to quality benchmarks for hospitals, and to support QI.[8] It captures data about all patients diagnosed with or treated for any type of cancer at CoC-accredited institutions, including patient demographics, tumor characteristics, treatment regimens, and cancer-related outcomes.[8] The NCDB includes patients who are initially diagnosed or treated at a non-CoC accredited hospital and subsequently received treatment at a CoC center, in which case, initial diagnostic and treatment information are retroactively captured.[9] Data are gathered by Certified Tumor Registrars and undergo extensive data integrity testing.[10] The NCDB captures greater than 70% of all new cancer diagnoses in the United States and is the largest cancer database in the world, with more than 34 million records at present.[8]

Another prominent clinical registry is the National Surgical Quality Improvement Program (NSQIP). NSQIP had its origins in the Veterans' Affairs (VA) health system, where it was created in response to a government mandate that outcomes in the VA system be compared with the private sector for quality assurance.[2] In the early 1990s, NSQIP began recording preoperative patient characteristics and outcomes for surgeries performed in the VA system.[11] From these data, risk-adjusted outcomes were calculated accounting for the differences in patient characteristics, allowing for comparison of hospital outcomes and identification of targets for improvement.[2,12] Following initiation of NSQIP, risk-adjusted outcomes across the VA system improved, a change attributed in large part to the program.[11]

Based on the success of NSQIP in the VA system, the program was extended to the private sector through a partnership with the ACS, initially in a 14-hospital trial study, and eventually to the private sector at large in 2005.[13] Since that time, the program, now titled "ACS NSQIP," has grown to more than 600 hospitals in 49 states within the United States and 9 other countries.[7] The ACS NSQIP data collection process is based on a sampling algorithm that identifies a subset of cases at participating sites. Trained Surgical Clinical Reviewers at each site abstract data from the medical record for included patients. These data are then aggregated and risk adjusted. Performance reports are provided to participating hospitals semiannually and include institutional outcomes benchmarked against national data (**Fig. 1**). In addition, a deidentified dataset is available to participating sites for research use.[7]

As interest in outcomes across the field of surgery has grown, NSQIP has expanded into collecting more disease-specific outcomes. Starting in 2011, NSQIP added the option to record operation-specific variables through procedure-targeted modules for hospitals that wish to measure more detailed outcomes for certain procedure types, such as colectomy, vascular surgery, pancreatectomy, or hepatectomy. In addition, separate QI programs have been launched by the ACS for special patient populations, including the Metabolic and Bariatric Surgery Accreditation and Quality Improvement Program and Trauma Quality Improvement Program.[7] In parallel with the development of NSQIP, other specialty societies also created their own registries, such as the Society of Vascular Surgery Vascular Quality Initiative and Society of Thoracic Surgery (STS) National Database.[14,15] At present, there are numerous clinical registries in the modern era that can assist in outcome measurement, QI, and research for a wide range of patients and diseases.

CLINICAL VERSUS ADMINISTRATIVE DATA—WHICH IS BETTER?

The ever-growing number of data sources, both clinical and administrative, can make it challenging to choose the appropriate data source to meet QI needs. Because of the cost and resources necessary to support a clinical registry, the use of administrative

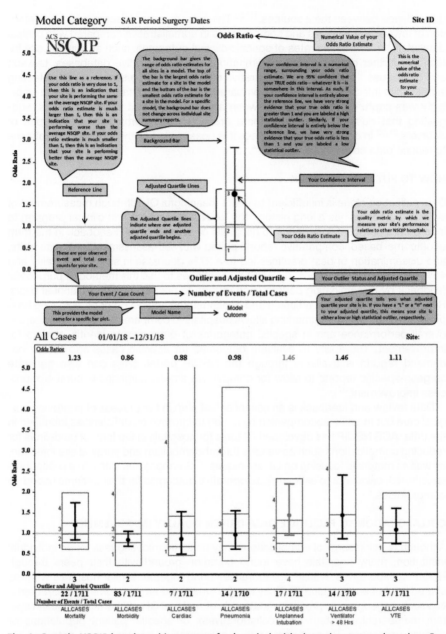

Fig. 1. Sample NSQIP benchmarking report for hospital with data element explanation. *Reproduced from* The American College of Surgeons Division of Research and Optimal Patient Care, with permission.

data in QI may be an appealing and cost-effective strategy for hospitals. However, the question remains whether data collected via payment charges are equivalent to those collected via clinical abstraction. Studies comparing detection of surgical complications in various clinical registries to administrative sources have found substantial discordance between the 2 sources.[16–29] The most common discrepancy was detection of fewer complications and comorbidities in administrative compared with clinical datasets.[20–22] Examining rates of specific clinical outcomes, such as surgical site infections, further demonstrates the limitations of administrative databases. Lawson and colleagues[30] found that administrative databases have a sensitivity for detecting surgical site infection of only 25% compared with clinical databases. However, mortality was captured comparably between administrative and clinical datasets, suggesting that despite differences, there are actionable items from both types of datasets.[31,32] In addition, in some cases it is possible to link the 2 types of databases to reduce data collection burden.[33,34]

HOW TO PUT DATA TO WORK

Data collection alone is insufficient to enact meaningful QI. Although measurement of surgical outcomes has a long history, the VA NSQIP was the first clinical program to incorporate purposeful feedback to hospitals on a large scale. Feedback in the form of outcome-based, comparative reports paired with self-assessment tools, site visits, and dissemination of best practices led to a 27% decrease in surgical mortality and 45% decrease in morbidity.[35] ACS NSQIP continues to use this method of purposeful feedback by disseminating performance reports to hospitals on a semiannual basis. Results are rigorously risk adjusted and benchmarked against other participating hospitals (see Fig. 1).[36] Benchmarking allows hospitals to compare themselves to peers in overall performance and in specific categories of outcomes to identify targets for improvement. The ability to evaluate outcomes for specific cases and review on-demand reports is available through the NSQIP portal. Sites can also generate surgeon-specific reports to allow for comparison among surgeons in pursuit of process improvement.[37]

Data review and feedback is an essential first step in the process of improving surgical care but must be accompanied by action to improve on deficiencies identified in the data. ACS NSQIP has developed QI tools for hospitals in the form of guidelines for reducing complications such as venous thromboembolism and surgical site infection, as well as materials focusing on QI techniques.[37] Surgeons can also use a procedure-specific risk calculator to estimate postoperative outcomes for their patients based on comorbidities.[9]

COLLABORATION TO FACILITATE DATA-DRIVEN QUALITY IMPROVEMENT

Although tackling surgical complications may be an intimidating task for an individual institution, many hospitals have found common ground with their peers through NSQIP collaboratives. NSQIP collaboratives bring together similar hospitals with the shared goal of encouraging QI. They can be structured around common characteristics such as geographic proximity (statewide or regional QI collaboratives), health system membership (system-wide collaboratives), or specific patient populations or disease processes. By participating in a collaborative, hospitals pool data and resources in pursuit of common QI goals. Sites with expertise in process improvement or success in certain outcomes can share knowledge and experience with other sites, allowing for quality to improve across multiple centers. Based on these principles, numerous collaboratives have demonstrated the ability to improve outcomes.

The Hepato-Pancreato-Biliary (HPB) NSQIP collaborative is an example of a disease-specific collaborative. It was established as a joint venture with the Americas Hepato-Pancreato-Biliary Association to address the high morbidity of HPB operations. It aims to leverage the QI potential of NSQIP through the pancreatectomy-

and hepatectomy-targeted data collection modules. More than 150 institutions currently share data for HPB operations across the collaborative and disease-specific outcomes, such as pancreatic leak or posthepatectomy liver failure, are targeted for improvement. More recently, the collaborative infrastructure and the NSQIP program have been used to launch a multicenter registry randomized controlled trial to study the effect of prophylaxis with a broad-spectrum penicillin compared with a second-generation cephalosporin on rates of surgical site infections after pancreato-duodenectomy.[38] By conducting the trial within the HPB collaborative, the existing network of hospitals was able to facilitate enrollment. In addition, the use of the pancreatectomy-targeted NSQIP dataset for data management removes significant logistical and financial barriers regarding prospective data collection.

Alternatively, the Illinois Surgical Quality Improvement Collaborative (ISQIC) is an example of a statewide collaborative that uses ACS NSQIP as the backbone for surgical QI. ISQIC was created to facilitate QI by providing education, mentorship, surgical coaching, and financial support to participating hospitals. The 55 hospitals that currently make up ISQIC encompass a diverse range of institutions, from small, rural hospitals to large, academic institutions. The major advantage in a collaboration such as ISQIC is through shared QI initiatives. Over its existence, ISQIC has launched initiatives related to reduction of venous thromboembolism, surgical site infection, and opioid reduction, among others. Other geographic regions have also demonstrated success in improving patient outcomes by regional collaboration.[39–42] Through a collaborative, hospitals with fewer resources or less experience in QI can learn from the experiences of those with expertise and tackle problems that are applicable to surgeons at any institution.

IMPACT OF REGISTRIES ON CLINICAL CARE

Utilization of ACS NSQIP and its associated QI tools to identify and address problems has been shown to improve patient care over time. An analysis of 116 participating hospitals over 3 years demonstrated that 66% of hospitals improved mortality and 82% of hospitals improved 30-day morbidity.[43] The greatest improvements were seen in low-performing hospitals, but high performers made improvements as well.[43] A more contemporary analysis of all participating NSQIP hospitals suggests that longer participation increases the magnitude of the benefit. Hospitals participating in NSQIP for at least 3 years had annual reductions of 0.8% in mortality, 3.1% in morbidity, and 2.6% in SSI, a larger improvement than seen in their less experienced peer hospitals.[44] In addition, participation in local and regional collaboratives allows for regional NSQIP audit of practice patterns and collaborative QI that has resulted in improvement in 30-day outcomes in multiple collaboratives.[39–42]

One of the primary methods by which patient safety and quality of care are monitored in cancer care is through CoC accreditation. In order to maintain CoC accreditation, hospitals are required to meet multiple program standards tracked in the NCDB.[45] These include fostering commitment to quality care and patient safety; maintaining the necessary administrative, institutional, and personnel resources to provide high-quality care; adhering to general and disease-specific clinical quality measures; demonstrating high quality in data collection; and engaging in education and outreach. In addition, CoC accredited institutions must engage in at least one QI initiative each year. In order to assist sites in this process, the CoC provides guidance on how to identify a target for improvement, implement an intervention, and monitor for improvement. Through these standards, the NCDB helps ensure high-quality cancer care and continued improvement.

ADMINISTRATIVE DATA IN QUALITY IMPROVEMENT

Although administrative databases can have limitations, they also can effectively drive QI initiatives. Well-known examples include the Patient Safety Indicators (PSIs) designed by AHRQ.[46,47] PSIs have been endorsed by the National Quality Forum, include surgery-specific measures, and have been used for comparison across hospitals and QI initiatives. Although PSIs have been shown to be potentially useful indicators to compare across hospitals, the accuracy of the measures can vary among PSI.[48,49] Another example is the Hospital Readmissions Reduction Program (HRRP), which as part of the Affordable Care Act, provided financial incentives to hospitals to reduce rates of readmission for certain medical procedures.[50] Although not directly addressing readmissions of surgical procedures, indirect effects were seen among surgical patients, with a decline in readmissions during the HRRP era.[43,51,52] Although it is not always possible to determine if a readmission is preventable based on coding data, HRRP has been used to initiate quality improvement. CMS has additionally used administrative data on selected quality measures to publicly report hospital performance and assign "star" ratings in an attempt for transparency and advancing QI.[4]

Privately purchased administrative databases such as Vizient or Premier have substantial potential to drive QI. Although the data inputs are primarily related to claims, these datasets integrate with the EMR and can be customized to fit the QI needs of the individual hospital.[5,6] These datasets also have the advantage of providing real-time feedback to clinicians and can track both outcomes and compliance to process measures. Data inputs can be aggregated into quality dashboards for review by committees to help with longitudinal tracking of quality efforts. Use of these dashboards has been shown to decrease surgical complications and length of stay.[53]

LIMITATIONS OF AVAILABLE DATASETS

Despite the great strides that have been—and continue to be—made in monitoring patient safety and enacting QI, there are several limitations of available datasets. First, most datasets lack customizability in content and timing of data collection. For logistical reasons, datasets generally collect the same variables for all patients and sites. Because data collection is coordinated from multiple sites and data quality must be validated, data are typically not available for a set period of time following clinical events. This reduces the utility of many datasets for customized QI initiatives or real-time outcomes monitoring. When planning to use a dataset for patient monitoring or QI, it is important to appreciate these limitations during project design and to set goals that can plausibly be achieved. As previously mentioned, certain datasets address some of these limitations by creating disease-specific cohorts to permit collection of more detailed data for specific procedures.

Another limitation of secondary datasets is data quality. Although nearly all national or regional datasets include some form of data quality assessment, erroneous and missing data are inevitable. This can occur due to errors in clinical diagnosis, documentation, or data abstraction. Prior studies have demonstrated that data quality in clinical registries is generally superior to administrative datasets, in part due to the robust checks in place on the data collection process.[30] For example, ensuring consistent data definitions for all variables, training and regularly testing data abstractors, and periodically auditing site data are methods used by ACS NSQIP.[54] Variables are also frequently reevaluated to reflect the current literature and best practices.[37]

Finally, due to data collection processes, administrative datasets have unique limitations. Because they are generally composed of billing encounters, it may not be possible to identify events, such as postoperative complications, that occurred outside a given encounter. Therefore, estimates of postoperative complications obtained from administrative data likely underreport the true incidence. Because administrative data are used to determine reimbursement, it is also possible that financial incentives affect data abstraction. For example, coding certain postoperative events such as sepsis or urinary tract infections elevates an encounter to a higher disease-related group. Because this results in increased reimbursement, hospitals may be incentivized to report these events at a higher rate than others that do not affect reimbursement. Given that payments for some hospitals are determined using alternate methodologies, this may also introduce bias in hospital comparisons.

THE QUALITY IMPROVEMENT FORMULA: INFRASTRUCTURE + DATA

Over nearly one hundred years of developing QI programs, the ACS has learned lessons about the necessary elements that must accompany data collection to improve surgical quality. First, a QI infrastructure is critical to the success of quality programs. Formalized case review, peer review, a quality control committee, and dedicated leadership in quality are integral to the successes of the trauma and bariatric programs developed with the ACS. Infrastructure modeled after these programs creates an organized flow of information to ensure adequate detection of problems and appropriate resource allocation to implement solutions and monitor progress. A variety of QI methodologies can be implemented within this framework, including Lean, Six Sigma, Plan-Do-Study-Act, and others.[55–59]

A second lesson learned from the ACS quality programs is the importance of a culture of safety and communication. Open communication from leadership and engagement of frontline workers can help create vertical integration of QI efforts for greater likelihood of success.[37] The teamwork and transparency generated by positive safety culture extends beyond QI; positive safety cultures have also been associated with improved patient outcomes.[60]

Finally, adapting QI efforts to the individual hospital is critical for success. Although datasets can be used to identify variation in practice patterns and opportunities for improved standardization, clinical protocols are not "one-size-fits-all" and must be adapted to the local environment. Enhanced recovery programs such as AHRQ Improving Surgical Care and Recovery can help provide the basic framework as a starting point for hospitals to standardize perioperative care. Identifying where guidelines must be adapted to fit the individual ethos of the hospital ensures greatest chance of implementation success.

Experience developing ACS quality programs such as trauma and bariatrics has highlighted the importance of infrastructure, culture, and standardized care as accompaniments to data-driven QI. Equally as evident is the inconsistency of implementation of these same principles across other areas of surgery not involved in a formal quality program. ACS Quality Verification was developed from lessons learned through experience with other ACS quality programs and is compiled into a manual about the necessary infrastructure, safety culture, care standardization, and best data practices to create a comprehensive quality program. The ideas in this program aim to counteract the siloing that occurs across surgical departments. This encourages organized information flow between leadership and frontline providers and creates a centralized quality structure that is nimble to respond to quality issues in surgery.

LOOKING TO THE FUTURE

Clinical registries have long been considered the gold standard in surgical QI. However, health care data are being generated at a staggering rate, introducing novel techniques to aggregate and use health care quality data. There is increasing interest in the use of app-based acquisition of clinical data from the electronic health record and machine learning algorithms for improving accuracy in diagnosis.[61] Wearable smart technology has also been introduced as a method to more effectively track postdischarge care.[62]

To expand the comprehensiveness of outcome measurement, interest is developing in expanding measurement beyond complications to outcomes that are important to patients. The importance of this is evident when considering surgical procedures with low rates of complications, in which differences in quality may not be appreciable using traditional outcomes such as death or readmission. Measuring what is important to the patient is the basis of patient-reported outcomes (PROs), which are defined as outcomes provided directly by the patient.[63] PROs are measured with psychometrically validated patient-completed questionnaires that record outcomes related to a particular health domain. At present, although PROs are widely used in research studies and institutional quality measurement, no national multispecialty registry has incorporated PROs. However, a pilot study is underway to assess the feasibility of collecting PROs from patients after surgery for use in the ACS NSQIP dataset. Although widespread inclusion of PROs in datasets is still well in the future, the potential opportunities are immense, allowing for assessment not just of complication rates but also the true experiences of patients following surgery.

In order to continue providing the best possible care to patients, it is important for surgical quality to remain nimble and use novel data in a thoughtful way. With increasingly larger quantities and newer forms of data collected on patients, there is also greater responsibility to protect patient privacy when using this data for QI.

SUMMARY

In summary, acquisition of data on clinical performance is essential to improve outcomes in surgery. Large, national datasets allow hospitals to monitor events involving patient safety and complications and facilitate QI development. National datasets also permit additional advantage of rigorous risk adjustment and ability to benchmark against peer hospitals or individual surgeons. Although clinical datasets are often preferable, administrative data also have potential for actionable QI. Hospitals should use whatever data resources may be available and be creative in combining data sources for the most clinically meaningful metrics. Although collection of data is essential in understanding the problems an individual hospital is facing, rigorous QI infrastructure is necessary to translate data to action and achieve sustained change.

CLINICS CARE POINTS

- Clinical performance data is essential to help surgeons improve outcomes.
- Large, national datasets can allow for identification of quality improvement issues. Benchmarking and rigorous risk adjustment are valuable tools to allow for peer comparison.
- Clinical data registries are ideal substrate for facilitation of quality improvement when available, however, administrative datasets can also be used for identification of quality and safety issues.
- Data collection is an important component of the quality improvement process, translation of data findings into action is critical for success and meaningful change.

DISCLOSURES

B.C. Brajcich and C.P. Fischer have no disclosures, financial or otherwise, to report. C.Y. Ko is the Director of the American College of Surgeons Division of Research and Optimal Patient Care.

REFERENCES

1. Neuhauser D. Ernest Amory Codman MD. Qual Saf Health Care 2002;11(1): 104–5.
2. Rodkey GV, Itani KM. Evaluation of healthcare quality: a tale of three giants. Am J Surg 2009;198(5 Suppl):S3–8.
3. Codman EA. The classic: a study in hospital efficiency: as demonstrated by the case report of first five years of private hospital. Clin Orthop Relat Res 2013; 471(6):1778–83.
4. Medicare Cf, Services M. CMS. gov. Baltimore (MD): Author; 2018.
5. Vizient I. Vizient. 2020. Available at: https://www.vizientinc.com/. Accessed April 22, 2020.
6. Health P. Premier health. 2020. Available at: https://www.premierhealth.com/. Accessed April 22, 2020.
7. American College of Surgeons. About ACS NSQIP. Available at: https://www.facs.org/quality-programs/acs-nsqip/about. Accessed April 15, 2020.
8. The American College of Surgeons. National cancer database. Available at: https://www.facs.org/quality-programs/cancer/ncdb. Accessed April 15, 2020.
9. Bilimoria KY, Stewart AK, Winchester DP, et al. The national cancer data base: a powerful initiative to improve cancer care in the United States. Ann Surg Oncol 2008;15(3):683–90.
10. Association NCR. Council on Certification. Available at: https://www.ncra-usa.org/CTR. Accessed April 15, 2020.
11. Itani KM. Fifteen years of the national surgical quality improvement program in review. Am J Surg 2009;198(5 Suppl):S9–18.
12. Fink AS. Adjusted or unadjusted outcomes. Am J Surg 2009;198(5 Suppl): S28–35.
13. Khuri SF, Henderson WG, Daley J, et al. Successful implementation of the department of veterans affairs' national surgical quality improvement program in the private sector: the patient safety in surgery study. Ann Surg 2008;248(2):329–36.
14. Society for vascular surgery. Vascular quality initiative. Available at: https://www.vqi.org/. Accessed April 15 , 2020.
15. The society of thoracic surgeons. STS National database. Available at: https://www.sts.org/registries-research-center/sts-national-database. Accessed April, 15 2020.
16. Ali-Mucheru MN, Seville MT, Miller V, et al. Postoperative surgical site infections: understanding the discordance between surveillance systems. Ann Surg 2020; 271(1):94–9.
17. Allen MS, Blackmon S, Nichols FC, et al. Comparison of two national databases for general thoracic surgery. Ann Thorac Surg 2015;100(4):1155–62.
18. Awad MI, Shuman AG, Montero PH, et al. Accuracy of administrative and clinical registry data in reporting postoperative complications after surgery for oral cavity squamous cell carcinoma. Head Neck 2015;37(6):851–61.
19. Bedard NA, Pugely AJ, McHugh MA, et al. Big data and total hip arthroplasty: how do large databases compare? J Arthroplasty 2018;33(1):41–5.e43.

20. Bensley RP, Yoshida S, Lo RC, et al. Accuracy of administrative data versus clinical data to evaluate carotid endarterectomy and carotid stenting. J Vasc Surg 2013;58(2):412–9.

21. Best WR, Khuri SF, Phelan M, et al. Identifying patient preoperative risk factors and postoperative adverse events in administrative databases: results from the department of veterans affairs national surgical quality improvement program. J Am Coll Surg 2002;194(3):257–66.

22. Borzecki AM, Cevasco M, Mull H, et al. Improving the identification of postoperative wound dehiscence missed by the Patient Safety Indicator algorithm. Am J Surg 2013;205(6):674–80.

23. Enomoto LM, Hollenbeak CS, Bhayani NH, et al. Measuring surgical quality: a national clinical registry versus administrative claims data. J Gastrointest Surg 2014;18(8):1416–22.

24. Koch CG, Li L, Hixson E, et al. What are the real rates of postoperative complications: elucidating inconsistencies between administrative and clinical data sources. J Am Coll Surg 2012;214(5):798–805.

25. Kulaylat AN, Engbrecht BW, Rocourt DV, et al. Measuring surgical site infections in children: comparing clinical, electronic, and administrative data. J Am Coll Surg 2016;222(5):823–30.

26. Lawson EH, Louie R, Zingmond DS, et al. A comparison of clinical registry versus administrative claims data for reporting of 30-day surgical complications. Ann Surg 2012;256(6):973–81.

27. Patterson JT, Sing D, Hansen EN, et al. The James A. Rand Young Investigator's award: administrative claims vs surgical registry: capturing outcomes in total joint arthroplasty. J Arthroplasty 2017;32(9):S11–7.

28. Steinberg SM, Popa MR, Michalek JA, et al. Comparison of risk adjustment methodologies in surgical quality improvement. Surgery 2008;144(4):662–9.

29. Davenport DL, Holsapple CW, Conigliaro J. Assessing surgical quality using administrative and clinical data sets: a direct comparison of the university health-system consortium clinical database and the national surgical quality improvement program data set. Am J Med Qual 2009;24(5):395–402.

30. Lawson EH, Zingmond DS, Hall BL, et al. Comparison between clinical registry and medicare claims data on the classification of hospital quality of surgical care. Ann Surg 2015;261(2):290–6.

31. Hall BL, Hirbe M, Waterman B, et al. Comparison of mortality risk adjustment using a clinical data algorithm (American College of Surgeons National Surgical Quality Improvement Program) and an administrative data algorithm (Solucient) at the case level within a single institution. J Am Coll Surg 2007;205(6):767–77.

32. O'Brien SM, Cohen DJ, Rumsfeld JS, et al. Variation in hospital risk–adjusted mortality rates following transcatheter aortic valve replacement in the United States: a report from the society of thoracic surgeons/American college of cardiology transcatheter valve therapy registry. Circ Cardiovasc Qual Outcomes 2016;9(5):560–5.

33. Beaulieu PA, Higgins JH, Dacey LJ, et al. Transforming administrative data into real-time information in the Department of Surgery. BMJ Qual Saf 2010;19(5):399–404.

34. Lawson EH, Louie R, Zingmond DS, et al. Using both clinical registry and administrative claims data to measure risk-adjusted surgical outcomes. Ann Surg 2016;263(1):50–7.

35. Khuri SF, Daley J, Henderson WG. The comparative assessment and improvement of quality of surgical care in the department of veterans affairs. Arch Surg 2002;137(1):20–7.
36. Cohen ME, Ko CY, Bilimoria KY, et al. Optimizing ACS NSQIP modeling for evaluation of surgical quality and risk: patient risk adjustment, procedure mix adjustment, shrinkage adjustment, and surgical focus. J Am Coll Surg 2013;217(2): 336–46.e331..
37. Ko CY, Hall BL, Hart AJ, et al. The American college of surgeons national surgical quality improvement program: achieving better and safer surgery. Jt Comm J Qual Patient Saf 2015;41(5):199–204.
38. ClinicalTrials.gov. Does cefoxitin or piperacillin-tazobactam prevent postoperative surgical site infections after pancreatoduodenectomy?. Available at: https://clinicaltrials.gov/ct2/show/NCT03269994. Accessed April 15, 2020.
39. Campbell DA, Englesbe MJ, Kubus JJ, et al. Accelerating the pace of surgical quality improvement: the power of hospital collaboration. Arch Surg 2010; 145(10):985–91.
40. Guillamondegui OD, Gunter OL, Hines L, et al. Using the national surgical quality improvement program and the Tennessee surgical quality collaborative to improve surgical outcomes. J Am Coll Surg 2012;214(4):709–14.
41. Vu JV, Collins SD, Seese E, et al. Evidence that a regional surgical collaborative can transform care: surgical site infection prevention practices for colectomy in Michigan. J Am Coll Surg 2018;226(1):91–9.
42. Vu JV, Englesbe MJ, Sheetz KH. Databases for surgical health services research: collaborative quality improvement programs. Surgery 2018;164(1):3–5.
43. Hall BL, Hamilton BH, Richards K, et al. Does surgical quality improve in the American college of surgeons national surgical quality improvement program: an evaluation of all participating hospitals. Ann Surg 2009;250(3):363–76.
44. Cohen ME, Liu Y, Ko CY, et al. Improved surgical outcomes for ACS NSQIP hospitals over time: evaluation of hospital cohorts with up to 8 years of participation. Ann Surg 2016;263(2):267–73.
45. Commission on Cancer. Optimal Resources for cancer care: 2020 standards. January 2020. Available at: https://www.facs.org/quality-programs/cancer/coc/standards/2020. Accessed April 15, 2020.
46. McDonald KM, Romano PS, Geppert J, et al. Measures of patient safety based on hospital administrative data-the patient safety indicators 2002. AHRQ Technical Reviews and Summaries. 2002. Report No.: 02-0038.
47. Miller MR, Elixhauser A, Zhan C, et al. Patient safety indicators: using administrative data to identify potential patient safety concerns. Health Serv Res 2001;36(6 Pt 2):110.
48. Kaafarani HM, Borzecki AM, Itani KM, et al. Validity of selected patient safety indicators: opportunities and concerns. J Am Coll Surg 2011;212(6):924–34.
49. Rivard PE, Luther SL, Christiansen CL, et al. Using patient safety indicators to estimate the impact of potential adverse events on outcomes. Med Care Res Rev 2008;65(1):67–87.
50. CMS. Hospital readmissions reduction program (HRRP). 2020. Available at: https://www.cms.gov/Medicare/Medicare-Fee-for-Service-Payment/AcuteInpatientPPS/Readmissions-Reduction-Program. Accessed April 17, 2020.
51. Borza T, Oerline MK, Skolarus TA, et al. Association of the hospital readmissions reduction program with surgical readmissions. JAMA Surg 2018;153(3):243–50.

52. Zuckerman RB, Sheingold SH, Orav EJ, et al. Readmissions, observation, and the hospital readmissions reduction program. N Engl J Med 2016;374(16): 1543–51.
53. Birdas TJ, Rozycki GF, Dunnington GL, et al. "Show me the data": A recipe for quality improvement success in an academic surgical department. J Am Coll Surg 2019;228(4):368–73.
54. Shiloach M, Frencher SK Jr, Steeger JE, et al. Toward robust information: data quality and inter-rater reliability in the American college of surgeons national surgical quality improvement program. J Am Coll Surg 2010;210(1):6–16.
55. Burgess N, Radnor Z. Evaluating Lean in healthcare. Int J Health Care Qual Assur 2013;26(3):220–35.
56. De Koning H, Verver JP, van den Heuvel J, et al. Lean six sigma in healthcare. J Healthc Qual 2006;28(2):4–11.
57. Kim CS, Spahlinger DA, Kin JM, et al. Lean health care: what can hospitals learn from a world-class automaker? J Hosp Med 2006;1(3):191–9.
58. Mazzocato P, Savage C, Brommels M, et al. Lean thinking in healthcare: a realist review of the literature. BMJ Qual Saf 2010;19(5):376–82.
59. Taylor MJ, McNicholas C, Nicolay C, et al. Systematic review of the application of the plan–do–study–act method to improve quality in healthcare. BMJ Qual Saf 2014;23(4):290–8.
60. Odell DD, Quinn CM, Matulewicz RS, et al. Association between hospital safety culture and surgical outcomes in a statewide surgical quality improvement collaborative. J Am Coll Surg 2019;229(2):175–83.
61. Obermeyer Z, Emanuel EJ. Predicting the future - big data, machine learning, and clinical medicine. N Engl J Med 2016;375(13):1216–9.
62. Appelboom G, Camacho E, Abraham ME, et al. Smart wearable body sensors for patient self-assessment and monitoring. Arch Public Health 2014;72(1):28.
63. Group. F-NBW. BEST (Biomarkers, EndpointS, and other Tools) resource. Silver spring (MD): food and drug administration. Bethesda (MD): National Institutes of Health; 2016.

The Economics of Patient Surgical Safety

Edwin Acevedo Jr, MD, MHA[a], Lindsay E. Kuo, MD, MBA[b],*

KEYWORDS

- Surgical safety • Surgical never events • Wrong-site surgery
- Retained foreign bodies • Surgical fires

KEY POINTS

- Adverse surgical events are a major cause of morbidity, mortality, and disability worldwide and remain a significant burden to patients, health care systems, and society.
- The financial cost of adverse surgical events to patients and health care systems is significant.
- Efforts have been made to reduce the incidence of surgical never events, but these events still occur.
- Sustained research in multiple aspects of prevention must continue to realize further gains in surgical safety.

INTRODUCTION

Surgery is an essential component of medical care. Nearly 17.2 million surgical procedures are being performed every year in the United States[1] and 234 million worldwide.[2] A myriad of advancements, such as sterilization and anesthesia administration, have fueled the wide delivery of surgery. Despite these innovations, surgery still has the potential to cause patient harm.

Adverse surgical events are a major cause of morbidity, mortality, and disability worldwide. The reported mortality rate following major surgery ranges from 0.5% to 5%; complications occur in up to 25% of inpatients.[3] More than 7 million patients experience an adverse event perioperatively each year, and 1 million patients die as a result. In the United States, the yearly costs associated with medical harm, such as subsequent health care expenses, lost income, and disability, are as high as $29 billion.[4]

[a] Temple University Lewis Katz School of Medicine, 3401 North. Broad Street, Philadelphia, PA 19140, USA; [b] Temple University Lewis Katz School of Medicine, 3401 North Broad Street Parkinson Pavilion, 4th, Fl, Philadelphia, PA 19140, USA
* Corresponding author.
E-mail address: Lindsay.kuo@tuhs.temple.edu
Twitter: @iamaceMD (E.A.); @lindsaykuo (L.E.K.)

Surg Clin N Am 101 (2021) 135–148
https://doi.org/10.1016/j.suc.2020.09.005
0039-6109/21/© 2020 Elsevier Inc. All rights reserved.
surgical.theclinics.com

At least one-half of the surgical harm is considered preventable.[3] To address preventable harm, the World Health Organization introduced the Surgical Safety Checklist more than 10 years ago. Other innovations, such as the standardization of preoperative antibiotic administration and thrombotic prophylaxis, have also contributed to a decrease in postoperative morbidity and mortality. Despite these measures, adverse surgical events remain a significant burden to patients and health care systems. In this article, we define patient surgical safety, discuss the attempts at risk reduction and the costs associated with safety failures, and provide an economic overview of the cost of reducing harm in surgical patients.

DEFINITION OF SURGICAL SAFETY

Health care–related harm is defined as an "harm arising from or associated with plans or actions taken during the provision of health care, rather than an underlying disease or injury (Available at: The Conceptual Framework for the International Classification for Patient Safety, World Health Organization, January 2009)." In the realm of surgery, harm can manifest in a number of ways, ranging from delayed diagnosis to postoperative complications and death. To address the wide potential for surgical harm, a number of quality metrics have been developed for every surgical subspecialty, at every phase of care, and in every setting.

A subset of preventable adverse events are considered serious reportable events (SREs), defined by the National Quality forum as "clearly identifiable and measurable," "usually preventable," and causing "death or loss of a body part, disability, or more than transient loss of a body function" (**Box 1**).[5] More commonly known as "never events," surgical SREs include wrong site, wrong procedure, and wrong patient surgery, and retained foreign bodies (RFBs). Other never events that can also occur in the perioperative setting include fires leading to burns, medication errors, and mismatched transfusions (**Table 1**). Although these events are rare, a 2013 publication by Mehtsun and colleagues[6] estimated that more than 4000 surgical SREs occur yearly, or 78.5 events weekly, in the United States.

Because of the preventable, consequential nature of SREs, there are multiple efforts to reduce their occurrence in the United States. Most states require public reporting of

---

Box 1
Criteria for Inclusion on the Never Event List

- *Unambiguous*—clear identifiable and measurable, and thus feasible to include in a reporting system;

- *Usually preventable*—recognizing that some events are not always avoidable given the complexity of health care;

- *Serious*—resulting in death or loss of a body part, disability, or more than a transient loss of a body function; and

- Any of the following:
  Adverse, and/or
  Indicative of a problem in a health care facility's safety systems, and/or
  Important for public credibility or public accountability.

From Eliminating Serious, Preventable, and Costly Medical Errors-Never Events. The Center of Medicare & Medicaid Services Website. https://www.cms.gov/newsroom/fact-sheets/eliminating-serious-preventable-and-costly-medical-errors-never-events. Published May 18, 2006. Accessed September 14, 2020.

Table 1
Current National Quality Safety Forum list of "never events"

Surgical events	Surgery or other invasive procedure performed on the wrong body part Surgery or other invasive procedure performed on the wrong patient Wrong surgical or other invasive procedure on a patient Unintended retention of a foreign object in a patient after surgery or other procedure Intraoperative or immediately post-operative death in an American Society of Anesthesiologists Class 1 patient
Product or device events	Patient death or serious injury associated with the use of contaminated drugs, devices or biologics provided by the health care facility Patient death or serious disability associated with the use or function of a device in patient care in which the device is used or functions other than as intended Patient death or serious disability associated with intravascular air embolism that occurs while being cared for in a health care facility
Patient protection events	Discharge or release of a patient or resident of any age who is unable to make decisions to other than an authorized person Patient death or serious disability associated with patient elopement (disappearance) Patient suicide, or attempted suicide resulting in serious disability, while being cared for in a health care facility
Care management events	Patient death or serious disability associated with a medication error Patient death or serious disability associated with unsafe administration of blood products Maternal death or serious disability associated with labor or delivery on a low-risk pregnancy while being cared for in a health care facility Death or serious injury of a neonate associated with labor or delivery in a low-risk setting Patient death or serious injury associated with a fall while being cared for in a health care facility Any stage 3, stage 4, or unstageable pressure ulcer acquired after admission or presentation to a health care facility Artificial insemination with the wrong donor sperm or wrong egg Patient death or serious disability resulting from the irretrievable loss of an irreplaceable biological specimen Patient death or serious disability resulting from failure to follow-up or communicate radiology test results
Environmental events	Patient or staff death or serious disability associated with an electric shock in the course of a patient care process in a health care setting Any incident in which a line designated for oxygen or gas to be delivered to a patient contains the wrong gas or is contaminated by toxic substances Patient or staff death or serious injury associated with a burn incurred from a patient care process in a health care setting

(continued on next page)

Table 1 (continued)	
	Patient death or serious injury associated with the use of restraints or bedrails while being cared for in a health care setting
Radiologic events	Death or serious injury of a patient or staff associated with introduction of a metallic object into the MRI area
Criminal events	Any instance of care ordered by or provided by someone impersonating a physician, nurse, pharmacist, or other licensed health care provider Abduction of a patient of any age Sexual assault on a patient within or on the grounds of a health care facility Death or significant injury or a patient or staff member resulting from a physical assault (ie, battery) that occurs within or on the grounds of a health care facility

Adapted from the List of SREs. National Quality Forum Website. http://www.qualityforum.org/Topics/SREs/List_of_SREs.aspx. Accessed September 14, 2020; with permission.

SREs. All never events are also considered "sentinel events" by the Joint Commission, which mandates root cause analysis following any sentinel event. In an effort to realign funding to focus on eliminating SREs, the Centers for Medicare and Medicaid Services has not paid for any care involving a preventable never event since 2009; many state and private insurers have followed suit.[7]

Next, we discuss 3 surgical never events and the associated costs of prevention and failure.

Wrong Site, Wrong Procedure, and Wrong Patient Events

WSPEs occur when surgery is performed on the wrong surgical site (eg, the right leg rather than the left leg), the wrong patient (ie, a patient undergoes an operation intended for a different patient), or wrong procedure is performed. WSPEs are overall rare, occurring in 1 out of 112,000 operations, but this number is likely much higher when including procedures occurring outside of the operating room.[7] Over a 1-year period between 2007 and 2008, there were 132 wrong site and wrong patient procedures in Colorado, occurring equally in operative and nonoperative settings.[8] A 2006 study estimated that there are 1300 to 2700 WSPEs annually in the United States.[9] WSPEs most commonly occur after orthopedic, general surgery, urologic, and neurosurgical procedures.[10]

Two tools were first introduced to reduce the likelihood of WSPEs. Surgical site marking—in which the operative surgeon clearly marks the operative location—was used as a means of preoperatively identifying the correct surgical site. However, this measure alone was an insufficient intervention.[7] Root cause analyses of wrong site surgery have identified a number of contributing factors, notably poor communication and missing documentation.[11] A list of system and process factors found to be causes of wrong site surgery can be found in **Table 2**. In an attempt to improve and standardize communication, the Joint Commission on Accreditation of Healthcare Organizations mandated the use of the universal protocol before all procedures, inside and outside the operating room.[12] The universal protocol consists of a preprocedural verification process, surgical site marking, and a preoperative "time out" to review the important aspects of the procedure with all participants. The time out is now generally performed as part of a more comprehensive surgical safety checklist.[11]

Table 2	
Causes of wrong-site, wrong-patient, wrong-procedure events	
System Factors	**Process Factors**
Lack of institutional controls or a formal system to verify the correct site of surgery	Inadequate patient assessment
	Inadequate care planning
Lack of a checklist to make sure every check was performed	Inadequate medical record review
	Miscommunication among members of the surgical team and the patient
Exclusion of certain surgical team members	
Reliance solely on the surgeon for determining the correct surgical site	More than 1 surgeon involved in the procedure
Unusual time pressures (eg, unplanned emergencies or a large volume of procedures)	Multiple procedures on multiple parts of a patient performed during a single operation
Pressures to reduce preoperative preparation time	Failure to include the patient and family or significant others when identifying the correct site
Procedures requiring unusual equipment or patient positioning	Failure to mark or clearly mark the correct operation site
Team competency and credentialing	
Availability of information	Incomplete or inaccurate communication among members of the surgical team
Organizational culture	
Orientation and training	Noncompliance with procedures
Staffing	Failure to recheck patient information before starting the operation
Environmental safety and security	
Continuum of care	
Patient characteristics, such as obesity or unusual anatomy, that require alterations in the usual positioning of the patient	

From Mulloy DF, Hughes RG. Wrong-Site Surgery: A Preventable Medical Error. In: Hughes RG, ed. Patient Safety and Quality: An Evidence-Based Handbook for Nurses (Prepared with support from the Robert Wood Johnson Foundation). AHRQ Publication No. 08-0043. Rockville, MD: Agency for Healthcare Research and Quality; March 2008.

Since widespread implementation of the universal protocol, there have been significant decrease in wrong site surgery.[12] Unfortunately, WSPEs still occur owing to breakdowns of the established checklist system. Time pressures, emergency surgery, physician distraction or fatigue, and the absence of a culture focused on patient safety may all lead to inattentive or cursory performance of the time out.[13] Further efforts to improve the communication, teamwork and a culture of patient safety will continue to decrease the occurrence of WSPEs.

Retained Foreign Body

RFBs or retained surgical items refer to surgical items or instruments unintentionally retained in the surgical site after skin closure. RFBs can have catastrophic implications for patients, leading to infections, reoperation, longer hospitalization or readmissions, and even death. RFBs occur as frequently as 1 out of 5500 operations, and the incidence is substantially higher in operations performed on open cavities.[14,15] Sponges are the most commonly retained item; surgical instruments are the second most common.[16,17]

Causes of RFBs are both case specific and related to the operating room environment. Emergency surgery, an unplanned change in the operation, increased body mass index, longer operative duration, and more major operations performed are risk factors for RFBs.[17] Incorrect instrument and sponge counts, shift changes during the case, as well as poor communication between surgical staff, also contribute.[12,16] Root cause analyses of these events, however, are inherently difficult to accomplish because many of the errors are not discovered immediately, making it impossible to recreate the causal chain in many cases.

The World Health Organization Surgical Safety Checklist includes ensuring a correct sponge and instrument count before the patient leaves the operating room.[4] Sponge and instrument counts alone, however, are insufficient; up to 88% of RFBs occur despite a reportedly accurate final count.[17] Additional methods have been used and technologies have been created to reduce the number of retained surgical instruments, such as use of selective radiographs, bar-coded sponges, and radiofrequency-tagged sponges.[18] A recent publication reported that after the implementation of a multidisciplinary approach to RFB prevention centered on training and education at a single institution, no RFBs occurred in more than 1300 days.[19] The most successful means of risk reduction may, in fact, be improved communication, teamwork, and organizational culture, as shown in **Table 3**.[20]

Surgical Fires

Surgical fires occur an estimated 550 to 650 times yearly in operating rooms in the United States.[19] Surgical fires occur when there is an ignition source (eg, electrosurgical units, electrocautery devices, lasers, light cords), fuel (eg, endotracheal tubes, alcohol-based preparatory solution, drapes and towels, or the patient's hair, skin, or tissue), and the presence of oxygen.[12,21] The risk of surgical fires increases with procedures involving the face and neck, such as tracheostomy, or when there an open oxygen source. Surgical fires can lead to disfiguring second- and third-degree burns and even death, and can be harmful to staff as well.

On root cause analysis of surgical fires, equipment issues, use of alcohol-based preparation solution, and provider behavior—such as starting the surgery before the preparation solution was dry—were noted to be contributing factors.[12] The American

Table 3		
Recommendations to reduce the incidence of RFBs		
Human Factors	**Leadership**	**Communication**
Provide team training	Prioritize a culture of safety	Verbally acknowledge
Address disruptive behavior	Conduct a proactive risk	removal of objects
Minimize distractions and	assessment and implement	Discuss removal of objects
interruptions	policies and procedures	during standardized
Account for objects inserted	based on the risk	debriefing
into the wound	assessment	Discuss the need for packing
Methodologically explore	Celebrate successes but also	removal during handoff
the surgical site before	encourage reporting of	Document verification of
closure	near misses	removal and integrity of
Verify integrity of objects		objects
upon removal		
Educate staff about risks of		
unintentionally retained		
foreign objects and risk		
reduction strategies		
Assess competency of		
personnel		

Adapted from Steelman VM, Shaw C, Shine L, et al. Unintentionally retained foreign objects: a descriptive study of 308 sentinel events and contributing factors. *Jt Comm J Qual Patient Saf.* 2019;45(4):249-258; with permission.

Society of Anesthesiologists Task Force on Operating Room Fires has created practice advisories to identify situations conducive to fire, decrease adverse events, and prevent their occurrences.[22] Additionally, the US Food and Drug Administration recommends that all health care staff should be trained to reduce surgical fires, including management of fires, fire drills, use of fire extinguishers, and evacuation procedures.[21] Specific recommendations are shown in **Box 2**. Interventions aimed at reducing surgical fires have been relatively successful and have reduced the incidence of surgical fires.[23] Nonetheless, these never events do occur, albeit at a low rate, and can lead to significant patient morbidity.

COST OF SURGICAL NEVER EVENTS

Costs associated with never events encompass a broad set of considerations, including the costs to the patient, costs to the health care system, and costs to society. There are additional nonfinancial economic consequences that must also be considered. In this section, we focus on the cost of surgical safety failures and discuss how failed interventions contribute to health care expenditures.

Cost to the Patient

Patients absorb the most significant costs when there is an event associated with surgical safety failure. There is significant morbidity, mortality, and disability associated with unsafe surgical practices. In a study of medical malpractice claims in the United States from 1990 to 2010, there were 9744 paid settlements and judgements for RFBs,

---

Box 2
Recommendations to reduce surgical fires

- *Fire risk assessment at the beginning of the surgical procedure.* The highest risk procedures involve supplemental oxygen and use of an ignition source near the oxygen (head, neck, or upper chest).

- Encourage communication among surgical team members.

- *Safe use and administration of oxidizers.* Evaluate if supplemental oxygen is needed. When available and appropriate, use a closed oxygen delivery system.

- *Safe use of any devices that serve as an ignition source.* Consider alternatives to using an ignition source if head/neck/chest surgery and if high concentrations of supplemental oxygen are being delivered. Inspect all instruments for evidence of insulation failure. Keep cautery instrument tips clean and free of char and tissue. Do not use monopolar electrosurgical units near other instruments and when not in use, place all devices in a designated area away from the patient, not on the patient or surgical drapes.

- *Safe use of items that may serve as a fuel source.* Allow for adequate drying time and prevent alcohol-based antiseptics from pooling during skin preparation. Use the appropriate size applicator. Be aware of drapes, plastics, and patient-related sources that can serve as a fuel.

- *Plan and practice how to manage a surgical fire.* Stop the main ignition source, extinguish the fire, remove all drapes and burning materials, and assess for smoldering materials. For airway fires, disconnect the patient from the breathing circuit and remove the endotracheal tube, then reestablish the airway once in a safe environment.

Data from Recommendations to Reduce Surgical Fires and Related Patient Injury: FDA Safety Communication. U.S. Food & Drug Administration Website. https://www.fda.gov/medical-devices/safety-communications/recommendations-reduce-surgical-fires-and-related-patient-injury-fda-safety-communication. Published May 29, 2018. Accessed September 14, 2020.

WSPEs.[6] Mortality occurred in 6.6% of patients, permanent injury in 32.9% of patients, and temporary injury in 59.2%.[6]

Adverse events also result in longer hospital stays and additional procedures. In a Dutch investigation into length of stay associated with adverse events, researchers found that patients who experienced an adverse event were hospitalized for 5.11 days longer than patients who did not.[24] In a landmark Canadian study investigating adverse events, patient care episodes—defined as all hospital care, long-term care and home care—were more than 2 weeks longer after hospital harm than when no harm occurred.[25] Although these studies do not focus solely on surgical never events, the potential for longer hospital stays and overall medical care following a surgical never event is significant.

There are also significant intangible costs to the patient when an event occurs as a result of a surgical safety failure. Pain, depression, anxiety, and stress caused by the trauma of unsafe surgical practices are easily identified, but very difficult to measure and assign value.[26] This emotional load is carried not just by the patient, but also by the patient's relatives.[26] Although the direct and indirect costs associated with medical care can be defined and calculated, intangible costs often lack the granularity that would enable them to be accurately enumerated. Nonetheless, these emotional aspects can greatly affect quality of life.

Last, there are the direct financial expenses stemming from the adverse event. These include copayments, deductibles, and coinsurance.[24] Copayments are direct out-of-pocket costs that patients must pay for every episode of care. When unsafe surgical practices lead to hospital readmissions, reintervention or additional outpatient follow-up appointments, patients may be responsible for copayments for each event. A deductible is the amount the insured patient must pay before any benefits of their insurance plan are payable. In most insurance plans, the insurance deductible is paid on an annual basis; some plans have separate deductibles for outpatient surgery and hospitalization. Patients experiencing a surgical never event may therefore be personally responsible for greater expenses if the care following a surgical never event spans more than 1 calendar year or occurs in different care settings. Finally, there is coinsurance, which is a fixed percentage of medical fees for which the insured is responsible. Most plans that include coinsurance have a stop-loss provision, which defines a maximum out-of-pocket liability that an insured patient would pay in a given year.[24] Despite the stop-loss provision, patients may still be responsible for significant financial liability when surgical safety is compromised. In a study looking at inpatient, outpatient, and drug payment claims for Medicare enrollees with secondary employer coverage, patients who experienced a preventable surgical safety failure had 52% higher inpatient hospital expenditures and 11% higher outpatient expenditures than patients who had not.[27] This translated to an average difference of $35,617 for 90-day expenditures, of which Medicare patients were directly responsible for an average $6998.[27]

Beyond the financial liability, patients also suffer significant opportunity costs, in the form of lost wages and productivity owing to the disability that may be caused by adverse surgical events. This includes wages lost owing to the inability to work, reduction in wages owing to absenteeism, and exhaustion of sick time, medical leave, and other employer-sponsored benefits. Furthermore, adverse events can lead to a loss of productivity, where patients are ineffective or inefficient at work owing to sickness.

Cost to the Health Care System

Not only do surgical never events impose a significant burden on patients and families, they can also generate considerable strain on health system finances via the provision of additional care and consumption additional resources. The exact costs of surgical never events, however, remain unclear, because this question has not been examined specifically. Instead, the published literature focuses on direct medical costs after a wide range of adverse events, such as medication errors, deep venous thrombosis, and nosocomial infections. Furthermore, the costing methodologies in the published literature on costs after adverse events vary from study to study. Regardless, the literature is illustrative of the potential financial impact of surgical never events on hospitals and health care systems.

The large-scale magnitude of the financial consequences of adverse events cannot be overstated. A 2012 study examining all medical errors that occurred in the United States in 1 year, including surgical never events, determined that medical errors led to $17 billion (USD) of subsequent medical costs.[28] Similarly, 2019 examination of adverse events in a single Canadian province summed the additional cost owing to adverse events to $1,088,330,376.[25] A 2004 study from the Netherlands determined that the total direct medical costs of preventable adverse events comprise 1% of the yearly national health care budget, primarily owing to excess length of stay.[29]

The higher costs stemming from adverse events are due both to the event itself and to additional care rendered after the index admission.[25] A 2019 study investigating costs in 1 Canadian province calculated the total incremental hospital care days attributable to adverse events to 407,696 days; the incremental patient care exposure days, which also include postdischarge care, totaled 661,646 days.[25] A 2017 Danish study of adverse events found that the costs of care for patients in a 1-year period after an adverse event were twice that of patients who did not experience an adverse event.[30] On a hospital level, the estimated 2009 cost of the hospital admission related to a RFB was greater than $60,000[18]; this number has surely increased over the decade since.

Who is responsible for these costs? In the United States, hospitals and health care systems are increasingly liable for expenses related to adverse events. In 2008, Medicare stopped reimbursing hospitals for care related to preventable complications and medical errors, including retained foreign objects after surgery. This change in reimbursement is now forcing health care systems to absorb the associated costs. The Affordable Care Act has continued to decrease federal reimbursement for failure to reach quality benchmarks, such as 30-day readmission rates. As such, hospitals will be required to improve the quality of the care provided or face penalties and/or increased expenses related to surgical safety failures.

Hospitals and health systems must also face the liability and medicolegal costs associated with surgical never events. Litigation stemming from RFB events in 2009 averaged $150,000 per payout.[18] Approximately 79% of wrong-site, wrong-procedure, wrong-patient ophthalmic surgery and 84% of orthopedic surgeries lead to malpractice awards.[10] For the estimated 4000 yearly surgical never events in the United States, health systems pay out $1.3 billion in medical liability payments.[6]

Cost to Society

The measurement of health benefits or harm to society is a key issue in health economic evaluations. In general, medical care directly produces health, which in turn generates "utility," which is the economic measurement of value. Healthy people allocate less time to sickness and therefore have more healthy days to increase their utility and usefulness to society. When an adverse event occurs during surgery, the utility of that patient to society decreases because of the patient's morbidity and disability. The patient may be absent from work or less productive when at work; some patients may become unemployed as a result of their disability. Based on short-term disability claims after medical errors in 2008 alone, 10 million days of productivity were lost.[31] Additionally, death after an adverse event leads to premature exit from the workforce. When factoring in the losses owing to death, the total economic costs nears $1 trillion yearly.[32]

There are additional intangible costs borne by society after an adverse event. Family members may become nonpaid caregivers to a patient, and their productivity in the workforce may decrease as a result. The negative impact on patients' and caregivers' quality of life cannot be quantified and can have enormous and lasting consequences. The surgical staff may experience significant emotional distress following a surgical never event, which can have downstream effects on a surgeon or staff member's ability to work effectively going forward.[33] The effects of a surgical never event are felt far and wide, and their true costs to society are unknown.

COSTS OF PREVENTION

Many interventions, programs, and initiatives have been developed to decrease harm and improve patient surgical safety. One widely adopted practice is the universal protocol, as discussed elsewhere in this article, which was developed in part to minimize the chance of WSPEs. The Surgical Safety Checklist, which incorporates the fire risk associated with operation into the preoperative time out, is another example. These protocols aim reduce the frequency and economic burden of surgical safety failures by improving quality and standardization.

Surgical never events are costly and, as a consequence, most hospitals have focused on improving quality to decrease the economic burden of unsafe surgical practices. Quality improvement efforts focus on process and quality metrics that can prevent wrong site surgery, retained surgical instruments, surgical fires, and other surgical postoperative morbidity. Implementing these changes can be expensive, and hospitals and health systems are likely to bear the responsibility for these sunk costs. Financial considerations may therefore be an obstacle to wider adoption of these best practices. Unfortunately, few studies have been performed examining the costs of quality improvement efforts, and even fewer examining the cost-effectiveness of these efforts in comparison to the cost of never events.[34]

One rare example of literature investigating the cost effectiveness of a quality intervention is a study published by Regenbogen and colleagues,[18] which compares the cost effectiveness of 3 alternatives to the standard counting process to address retained surgical sponges. This complex decision analysis incorporated information on the frequency of retained surgical sponges and the cost estimates for various strategies to identify a retained sponge: (1) no sponge counting, (2) standard sponge counting, (3) universal x-ray films without counting, (4) universal x-ray films with counting, (5) selective x-ray films for high-risk operations, (6) bar-coded sponges, and (7) radiofrequency sponge systems. The incidence of retained sponges without any counting is 67 per 100,000 operations, and standard counting alone reduces the frequency of these events to 12 per 100,000. Bar-coded sponges were the most cost effective, reducing the frequency of retained sponges to an estimated 1.7 per 100,000 and costing $95,000 for each retained sponge prevented. Radiofrequency sponge systems were equally effective but more costly, at $720,000 per retained sponge avoided, and all forms of x-ray were both less effective and more costly.[18]

Few other studies provide this comparative cost information, even for more common adverse events. This gap in knowledge is an area in need of exploration, because health systems need to know cost of safety improvements.[34] Furthermore, cost alone may not be the only factor in decision making. Regenbogen and colleagues[18] acknowledge that hospitals may choose any of the sponge tracking methods despite awareness of varying cost effectiveness. Every hospital and health system will have a different willingness to pay to prevent these events. External factors affecting these decisions include the local regulatory environment, the ease of use of each system, and the preferences of the staff inside the operating room itself.[18]

The ability of an individual hospital or an entire health system to adopt preventative measures varies. The Mayo Clinic implemented "Mayo Clinic Patient Safety Essentials" throughout all health system sites, and reported that implementation is "simple in some instances but in others requires a diffusion process equipped with project managers, systems engineers, communications experts, clinical experts, and the oversight of a high-level champion."[35] Many hospitals or health system may not have the resources to commit to complex, wide-reaching change, no matter how desirable the outcome. And, importantly, although the Mayo Clinic reduced their surgical never event frequency after the introduction of this program, these events still occur.[35]

Why do surgical never events still happen despite these efforts? New technologies have been developed to further decrease the likelihood of human error, but no hospital has reported zero never events. Many studies have commented on the importance of a culture in which employee knowledge, beliefs, and attitudes are focused on patient safety. Developing a culture of safety is a crucial feature in many quality improvement and patient safety efforts.[36] Studies examining safety culture variables and adverse clinical events found that a more positive patient safety culture is associated with decreased readmissions and fewer patient safety events.[37,38] Hiring practices, onboarding programs, and performance management programs can all impact an organization's safety climate.[39] To further decrease the incidence of surgical never events, hospitals must continue to invest in an institutional culture that prioritizes patient safety.

The cost of implementing these safety initiatives to improve the safety of surgery is the cost of prevention. Few studies have compared the prevention costs associated with quality improvement and safety initiatives to the costs of safety failures. But, by developing a culture of safety within an organization, safety is prioritized, which enables quality improvement efforts. Together, implementing best practices, quality improvement strategies, and cost-effective interventions can aid in reducing the never events. The costs of harm dwarf these actionable efforts to prevent adverse events.

SUMMARY

Safe surgical practice is a priority for surgeons and health care systems owing to the high costs associated with adverse events. Wrong site, wrong patient, wrong procedure surgery, retained surgical instruments, surgical fires, and postoperative morbidity account for a large amount of health care expenditures in the United States. Not only do these events lead to increased resource use and other costs to society, these errors contribute to significant morbidity, mortality, and disability, which directly affects the lives of the patients and their loved ones. The true cost of failure is unquantifiable. Although many innovations ranging from checklists to radiofrequency technology have been developed to eliminate surgical never events, these failures in safety still occur. Research into the cost effectiveness of preventative measures must continue to inform organizational decision making. Hospitals and health systems must work to grow and prioritize a culture of patient safety. There is no one-size-fits-all approach to this problem; instead, we must all work together to eradicate these never events.

CLINICS CARE POINTS

- System and process factors can contribute to never events.
- Human factors, including culture and communication, can reduce the likelihood of never events.

DISCLOSURE

The authors have nothing to disclose.

REFERENCES

1. Mathias J. AHRQ releases stats on outpatient, inpatient surgeries 2017. Available at: https://www.ormanager.com/briefs/ahrq-releases-stats-on-outpatient-inpatient-surgeries/. Accessed July 3, 2020.
2. Weiser TG, Regenbogen SE, Thompson KD, et al. An estimation of the global volume of surgery: a modelling strategy based on available data. Lancet 2008;372(9633):139–44.
3. World health organization. patient safety. Available at: https://www.who.int/patientsafety/topics/safe-surgery/en/. Accessed May 4, 2020.
4. National quality forum. List of SREs. Available at: http://www.qualityforum.org/Topics/SREs/List_of_SREs.aspx. Accessed May 4, 2020.
5. U.S. Centers for Medicare and Medicaid services. Eliminating serious, preventable, and costly medical errors - never events. Available at: https://www.cms.gov/newsroom/fact-sheets/eliminating-serious-preventable-and-costly-medical-errors-never-events. Accessed April 30, 2020.
6. Mehtsun W, Ibrahim AM, Diener-west M, et al. Surgical never events in the United. Surgery 2013;153(4):465–72.
7. Patient safety network. Wrong-site, wrong-procedure, and wrong-patient surgery. Patient safety primer. Available at: https://www.psnet.ahrq.gov/primer/wrong-site-wrong-procedure-and-wrong-patient-surgery#. Accessed May 4, 2020.
8. Stahel PF, Sabel AL, Victoroff MS, et al. Wrong-site and wrong-patient procedures in the universal protocol era. JAMA Surg 2010;145(10):978–84.
9. Seiden SC, Barach P. Wrong-side/wrong-site, wrong-procedure, and wrong-patient adverse events. JAMA Surg 2006;141(9):931–9.
10. Mulloy DF, Hughes RG. Wrong-site surgery - a preventable medical error causes and consequences of wrong-site surgery. In: Hughes R, editor. Patient safety and quality: an evidence-based handbook for nurses. Rockville (MD): Agency for Healthcare Research and Quality; 2008.
11. Haynes AB, Weiser TG, Berry WR, et al. A Surgical safety checklist to reduce morbidity and mortality in a global population. N Engl J Med 2009;360(5):491–9.
12. Hempel S, Maggard-Gibbons M, Nguyen D, et al. Wrong-site surgery, retained surgical items, and surgical fires: A systematic review of surgical never events. JAMA Surg 2015;150(8):796–805.
13. Health Research & Educational Trust and Joint Commission Center for Transforming Healthcare. Reducing the risks of wrong-site surgery: safety practices from the joint commission center for transforming healthcare project. Chicago (IL): Health Research & Educational Trust; 2014. Available at: www.hpoe.org.
14. Hariharan D, Lobo DN. Retained surgical sponges, needles and instruments. Ann R Coll Surg Engl 2013;95(2):87–92.
15. Cima RR, Kollengode A, Garnatz J, et al. Incidence and characteristics of potential and actual retained foreign object events in surgical patients. J Am Coll Surg 2008;207(1):80–7.
16. Williams TL, Tung DK, Steelman VM, et al. Retained surgical sponges : findings from incident reports and a cost-benefit analysis of radiofrequency technology. J Am Coll Surg 2014;219(3):354–64.
17. Gawande AA, Studdert DM, Orav EJ, et al. Risk factors for retained instruments and sponges after surgery. N Engl J Med 2003;348(3):229–35.

18. Regenbogen SE, Greenberg C, Resch S, et al. Prevention of retained surgical sponges: a decision-analytic model predicting relative cost-effectiveness. Surgery 2009;145(5):527–35.
19. Duggan EG, Fernandez J, Saulan MM, et al. 1,300 days and counting: a risk model approach to preventing retained foreign objects (RFOs). Jt Comm J Qual Patient Saf 2018;44(5):260–9.
20. Steelman VM, Shaw C, Shine L, et al. Unintentionally retained foreign objects: a descriptive study of 308 sentinel events and contributing factors. Jt Comm J Qual Patient Saf 2019;45(4):249–58.
21. U.S. Food and drug administration. Recommendations to reduce surgical fires and related patient injury: FDA safety communication. Available at: https://www.fda.gov/medical-devices/safety-communications/recommendations-reduce-surgical-fires-and-related-patient-injury-fda-safety-communication. Accessed April 23, 2020.
22. Apfelbaum J, Caplan R, Barker S, et al. Practice advisory for the prevention and management of operating room fires. Anesthesiology 2008;108(5):786–801.
23. Bruley ME, Arnold TV, Finley E, et al. Surgical fires: decreasing incidence relies on continued prevention efforts. Pa Patient Saf Advis 2018;15(2):1–12.
24. Shi L, Singh D. Cost, access, and quality. In: Essentials of the U.S. health care system. 4th edition. Burlington (MA): Jones & Bartlett Learning; 2017. p. 135–66.
25. Tessier L, Guilcher SJ, Bai YQ, et al. The impact of hospital harm on length of stay, costs of care, and length of person-centered episodes of care: a retrospective cohort study. CMAJ 2019;191:879–85.
26. Kobiela J, Kobiela P. Emotional aspects of never events. JAMA Surg 2016; 151(1):95–6.
27. Encinosa WE, Hellinger FJ. What Happens After a Patient Safety Event? Medical expenditures and outcomes in Medicare. Rockville (MD): Agency for Healthcare Research and Quality; 2005.
28. de Rezende BA, Or Z, Com-ruelle L, et al. Economic evaluation in patient safety: a literature review of methods. BMJ Qual Saf 2012;21:457–65.
29. Hoonhout LHF, Bruijne MCD, Wagner C, et al. Direct medical costs of adverse events in Dutch hospitals. BMC Health Serv Res 2009;9(27):1–10.
30. Kjellberg J, Wolf RT, Kruse M, et al. Costs associated with adverse events among acute patients. BMC Health Serv Res 2017;17(651):1–7.
31. Shreve J, Van Den Bos J, Gray T, et al. The economic measurement of medical errors. Schaumburg, IL: Society of Actuaries; 2010. p. 270–4.
32. Andel C, Davidow SL, Hollander M, et al. The economics of health care quality and medical errors. J Health Care Finance 2012;39(1):39–50.
33. Serou N, Sahota L, Husband AK, et al. Systematic review of psychological , emotional and behavioural impacts of surgical incidents on operating theatre staff. BJS Open 2017;1:106–13.
34. Etchells E, Koo M, Daneman N, et al. Comparative economic analyses of patient safety improvement strategies in acute care: a systematic review. BMJ Qual Saf 2012;21:448–56.
35. Morganthaler T, Harper CM, "Getting Rid of 'Never Events' in Hospitals." Harvard Business Review, October 20, 2015. Available at: https://hbr.org/2015/10/getting-rid-of-never-events-in-hospitals.
36. Weaver S, Lubomski L, Wilson R, et al. Promoting a culture of safety as a patient safety strategy: a systematic review. Ann Intern Med 2013;158(5):369–74.
37. Mardon R, Khanna K, Sorra J, et al. Exploring relationships between hospital patient safety culture and adverse events. J Patient Saf 2010;6(4):226–32.

38. Hansen LO, Mark V, Singer SJ. Perceptions of hospital safety climate and incidence of readmission. Health Serv Res 2011;46(2):596–616.
39. Society for human resource management. Understanding and developing organizational culture. Available at: https://www.shrm.org/resourcesandtools/tools-and-samples/toolkits/pages/understandinganddevelopingorganizationalculture.aspx. Accessed May 6, 2020.

The Trainee's Role in Patient Safety

Training Residents and Medical Students in Surgical Patient Safety

Swara Bajpai, MD[a], Brenessa Lindeman, MD, MEHP[b],*

KEYWORDS

- Residents • Trainees • Medical students • Nontechnical skills • Simulation
- WHO Curriculum guide

KEY POINTS

- Many adverse events affecting patient safety occur in the perioperative setting and are often related to the overall health system, safety culture, and cohesiveness of teams.
- Medical school and surgical residency curricula must transition from the traditional sole emphasis on medical and operative knowledge to development of nontechnical skills such as effective leadership, communication, transition of care, and teamwork.
- General guidance in formalizing a patient safety curriculum for medical students has been developed by the World Health Organization.
- Systematic surgical residency training in patient safety is important and recommended by many national organizations such as the American College of Surgeons and Accreditation Council for Graduate Medical Education, yet remains inconsistent and incomplete.

INTRODUCTION

Much evidence shows that almost half of adverse events occur after surgical or other invasive procedures.[1] Although adverse events related to surgery were traditionally thought to be related to the skills of the surgeon, complexity of the procedure, and the comorbidities of the patient, it is now known that these events are associated with many other factors such as the design of the specific health care system, elements of teamwork, and organizational culture,[2–4] which means that medical school and surgical residency curricula need to shift from the traditional emphasis on solely teaching medical and operative knowledge to a more holistic approach including

---

[a] Department of Surgery, 1808 7th Avenue South, BDB 202, Birmingham, AL 35294, USA;
[b] Endocrine Surgery, General Surgery, Department of Surgical Oncology, BDB 603, Birmingham, AL, USA
* Corresponding author. Department of Surgery, 1808 7th Avenue South, BDB 506, Birmingham, AL 35294.
E-mail address: blindeman@uabmc.edu

Surg Clin N Am 101 (2021) 149–160
https://doi.org/10.1016/j.suc.2020.09.007
0039-6109/21/© 2020 Elsevier Inc. All rights reserved.

elements of leadership development, improving teamwork skills, and fostering a culture that encourages recognition of and learning from errors.[5]

NATURE OF THE PROBLEM

Creating a culture of safety, closing communication gaps, and ensuring appropriate transition of care have all been identified as key factors in patient safety and error reduction, especially in the perioperative setting.[5]

THE SAFETY CULTURE

The Patient Safety Systems chapter of The Joint Commission accreditation manuals defines safety culture as the "product of individual and group beliefs, values, attitudes, perceptions, competencies, and patterns of behavior that determine the organization's commitment to quality and patient safety."[6] There is generally noteworthy variability in perceptions of perioperative safety culture based on professional roles and level of training, and as trainees are one of the front-line groups responsible for much direct patient care, it is imperative they are inculcated into this culture early on.

One research group examined safety culture at a tertiary care hospital by surveying 431 perioperative health care workers including anesthesia and surgery attendings and residents, nurses, and technicians. The domains of safety culture with the highest average positive scores were teamwork, organizational learning, and improvement. Domains with the lowest scores were feedback, communication about errors, and transition of care. Surgery attendings perceived the strongest safety climate overall, whereas nurses and surgical technicians perceived significantly worse safety culture, suggesting a hierarchical influence.[7] Putnam and colleagues has shown that despite an existing online patient safety curriculum, surgical residents continued to perceive the perioperative environment as more unsafe than attending surgeons, anesthesiologists, and other direct care providers who underwent an additional series of operative safety workshops. Resident scores were lower in their perceptions of safety culture, teamwork, and ability to speak up.[1] This serves as an opportunity to further identify the concerns of this group on the front lines of care and work to address them.

COMMUNICATION AND HANDOFFS

Communication breakdowns are among the most frequent contributors to adverse events, including in the perioperative setting, and reduction in these events can both substantially improve patient safety and reduce errors.[8] In an observational study of 48 surgical cases, Lingard and colleagues identified more than 400 procedurally relevant communication events and classified 30% of them as "failures." There is a global vulnerability in this setting to communication mishaps, with information loss occurring at every point from the patient's first surgical consultation to care in the recovery room.[9]

Communication often involves multiple agents, from attendings to trainees to ancillary staff.[9] A study of 60 surgical cases found that attending surgeons followed by surgical residents are the agents most frequently involved in these serious communication breakdowns. Uncertainty about roles, responsibilities, and leadership was common, occurring in at least 58% of cases.[2]

Handoffs and transfers in care are especially vulnerable to communication breakdown.[2,8,10] Approximately 40% of communication breakdowns occur in transition of care between providers.[2] Likewise, potentially preventable events are strongly associated with coverage by a physician from another team, likely secondary to incomplete handoff of patients.[11] It has been reported that level of communication and collaboration between surgical attendings, followed by those between residents, substantially correlate with risk-adjusted morbidity. This suggests a hierarchical importance of their roles, perhaps of decision-making in the clinical setting, but nonetheless that improving communication among attendings and residents can reduce patient morbidity.[12] The abovementioned results suggest we prioritize the development of standardized handoffs, transfer protocols, and communication triggers that apply to all staff, including trainees.[2] Traditionally, residents have ensured continuity of care by working longer shifts, minimizing the transfer of responsibilities to other providers. The 80-hour work week and other regulatory requirements have placed added pressure on trainees for workflow efficiency, making standardization of such processes even more important.[10]

Despite work hour restrictions, residents still struggle with workload, with more than half of respondents in a study conducted by Mundschenk and colleagues[13] stating they did not prepare for a surgical case because of other task requirements, exhaustion, or postcall status. With respect to patient safety, although 98% of trainees agreed that one of the most important steps in preparation for surgery is review of the patient's medical record, only 30% thought they were very prepared when asked to rate their patient-specific preparation. Most respondents thought they only "sometimes" or "rarely" had enough time to prepare for a case. This, not surprisingly, translated into poor transition of care in the postoperative setting. When rating the quality of their patient handoffs, only 24.2% of respondents thought they were comprehensive with regard to patient's medical history and operative course.[13]

Should residents hold themselves accountable for being as prepared as possible or should educators? In order to develop comprehensive training programs, the answer should be both. Whereas technical skill and surgical knowledge should certainly be emphasized in residency training, so should impact of thorough preparation and appropriate communication on patient safety and overall outcome. The importance of such should be instilled early on so that trainees proceed with only the best habits, and ideally this should begin in medical school.

STARTING IN MEDICAL SCHOOL: WHAT MEDICAL STUDENTS NEED TO KNOW ABOUT PATIENT SAFETY

Patient safety education is required learning particularly during the foundational years of medical education. Being aware that errors occur is not enough. The ideal practitioner integrates patient safety concepts into all areas of their practice. As future physicians and leaders, medical students must be aware of the multiple factors that influence health care outcomes and learn how to reduce opportunities for errors.[14] Students can begin to learn practical lessons about safety as soon as they enter clinical rotations, as are often best taught through examples in the wards.[14]

The case for training students in patient safety was first recognized in the Institute of Medicine report To Err is Human,[5] but only started to gather momentum nearly a decade later.[14] To address the gap, the Australian Patient Safety Education Framework[11] published an evidence-based description of the knowledge, skills, and behaviors required by all health care workers.[15] In 2009, The World Health Organization (WHO) World Alliance for Patient Safety acted further and used these guidelines in sponsoring the development of The WHO Patient Safety Curriculum Guide for medical schools worldwide.[14] The final guide was produced after collection of validity evidence by a worldwide panel of medical educators and patient safety experts and is readily available online for free download.[16] See **Box 1** for a complete list of topics covered.

Box 1
Topics in the World Health Organization curriculum guide

1. What is patient safety?
2. What are human factors, and why are they important to patient safety?
3. Understanding systems and the impact of complexity on| patient care
4. Being an effective team player
5. Understanding and learning from errors
6. Understanding and managing clinical risk
7. Introduction to quality improvement methods
8. Engaging with patients and carers
9. Minimizing infection through improved infection control
10. Patient safety and invasive procedures
11. Improving medication safety

Data from World Health Organization. Patient Safety Curriculum Guide for Medical Schools. Geneva, Switzerland: World Health Organization; 2009.

Topics are designed to either be integrated into existing didactics or introduced as stand-alone modules through panels, small group discussion sessions, or simulation exercises.[14]

The Curriculum Guide

Patient safety is a complex topic that includes new areas of focus sometimes unfamiliar to practitioners such as human factors, systems thinking, teamwork, root cause analysis, risk reduction, and quality improvement methods. Each should be included in developing a patient safety curriculum. Human factors is the science of the interrelationship between humans, their tools, and the environment. Students need to understand how human factors can contribute to adverse events and errors, as well as how the human–system interface can be improved by changing the design of the system and simplifying processes. This involves standardizing procedures, providing backup to human failures, improving communication, redesigning equipment, and propagating awareness of behavioral, organizational, and technological limitations that contribute to error.[3]

Students should be introduced to the concept that a health care system is not one, but many systems that make up a complex web of organizations, departments, units, and services that facilitate relationships between patients, caretakers, health care providers, support staff, administrators, bureaucrats, and economists. Medical students need to understand that although an individual provider can do their best in caring for patients, they will not be able to achieve safe and quality service alone. This is because patients depend on a system of care,[3] and application of lessons learned from other industries related to systems thinking can help to optimize outcomes for all stakeholders that are part of the system.

Medical students' thorough understanding of teamwork involves appreciating the benefits of multidisciplinary teams and how they can improve care and reduce errors. By witnessing effective teams at work, students will be able to appreciate the importance of communication as well as collaboration on decision-making and optimizing patient care. More importantly, they may be able to grasp how miscommunication between team members can be associated with delays in care, or worse yet, dangerous errors. This topic should present the underlying knowledge and opportunity for practice required to become an effective team member.[3]

Understanding root cause analysis is necessary for appreciating how design of systems and other factors contribute to errors in the health care system. Medical students need to understand how weak points of a system can lead to mistakes in order to develop awareness, learn when to anticipate system breakdowns, and prevent them from happening. An understanding of health care errors also provides the basis for making improvements and implementing effective reporting systems. Students should learn that a systems approach to errors is better than a person approach, which means prioritizing and understanding factors involved over seeking blame.[3,17]

Finally, quality improvement is a concept students should learn in order to be equipped with the tools to facilitate improvement in their own practice as well as the system they will one day work in. These include ability to identify and measure problems, develop interventions, and test them. This solidifies skills of identifying, examining, and understanding the step by step processes underlying successful health care delivery compared with failures. The key is grasping how aspects of care are connected and measurable.[3]

Teaching Patient Safety as It Pertains to Surgery

Although the abovementioned topics are all important to understanding patient safety across the spectrum of health care, a portion of the curriculum must be dedicated to care processes related to surgery and other invasive procedures given the high risks associated with these areas (**Box 1**, Topic 10). **Box 2** describes knowledge and performance objectives that are recommended to be covered by The WHO Curriculum Guide.[3] The guide was written to assist students in understanding how previously mentioned principles such as teamwork and standardization can support minimization of adverse events associated with invasive procedures.[3]

Observe and Practice Operating Room Techniques that Reduce Risks and Errors

Although they often cannot contribute to technical performance of a procedure, one area in which students can contribute greatly is in enhancing patient safety. They will be able to witness elements that can make or break a team, such as quality of leadership, communication intraoperatively and during handoffs, and history taking. If possible, students should[3]

Box 2
Knowledge and performance requirements in patient safety for medical students

Knowledge Requirements
- The main types of adverse events associated with surgical and invasive procedures care
- The verification processes for improving surgical and invasive procedures care

Performance Requirements
- Follow a verification process to eliminate wrong patient, wrong side, and wrong procedure
- Practice operating room techniques that reduce risks and errors (time-out, briefings, debriefings, stating concerns)
- Participate in an educational process for reviewing surgical and invasive procedures mortality and morbidity.

Data from World Health Organization. Patient Safety Curriculum Guide for Medical Schools. Geneva, Switzerland: World Health Organization; 2009.

- Identify the main protocols used in a particular surgical unit
- Understand how guidelines were developed and why they are necessary
- Identify the steps in the verification process including selection of the right patient, right site, and right procedure
- Identify how conflicts are resolved in the team
- Ask questions when appropriate
- State intentions clearly:
  ○ Students should practice declaring intentions and seek feedback before deviating from the norm, alerting the rest of the team about planned actions that are not routine
- Participate in team briefings and debriefings
- Observe and record the processes designed to keep the patient safe
- Evaluate their own contributions and ability to communicate patient status and care plans

Participate in an Educational Process for Reviewing Surgical Mortality and Morbidity

Most hospitals where surgery is performed will have a well-established confidential peer review system for discussing difficult cases, errors, and ethical dilemmas and serve as the main method for retrospection and future improvements. Because patient safety is a relatively new discipline, many of these meetings have yet to adopt a systems-based (rather than person-focused) approach. When meetings adopt a punitive attitude during discussions about errors, they are often closed to other members of the operating team. However, these mortality and morbidity meetings are excellent places to learn about error prevention. Medical students should try to attend if appropriate and observe to see how basic patient safety principles are demonstrated.[3]

A Note on Teaching Ethics

Participation in patient safety is one concrete expression of a foundational principle of medical ethics: do no harm. Thus, teaching concepts of patient safety go hand-in-hand with teaching principles of medical ethics. By 1990, medical ethics had become an integral part of the core curriculum in most American medical schools as part of an effort to develop students' values, perspectives, and interpersonal skills for the practice of medicine. One of the principle recommendations for undergraduate medical education is that new graduates should be inculcated with attributes appropriate to future responsibilities to their patients, colleagues, and society in general.[18]

As with patient safety, the ethical aspects of clinical decision-making should be made explicit during clinical teaching and example setting.[19] It is important to recognize the influence of the hidden curriculum, which likely affects students' ethical development more than the formal curriculum. Evidence has shown students to be more profoundly affected by role models than by formal coursework, and positive examples in the environment have the potential to counter the negative influence of cynical physician behavior.[18,19] This same principle can be applied to teaching patient safety. It is hoped that exceptional care with positive outcomes will serve as inspiration, countering examples of inadequate performance and poor outcomes.

PATIENT SAFETY IN RESIDENCY
Pitfalls

Surgical resident education is a constantly evolving field.[20] One pitfall is that training in technical skill and operative knowledge can become the only priorities, to the detriment of all other areas. But many factors influence surgical outcomes. As understanding of patient safety grows, there is increasing recognition of a surgeon's impact on outcomes that have a nontechnical basis. Specifically, safety experts stress that practitioners' interactions with each other (as a team) and with their environment (as a system) are critical determinants of error.[2] Attention must be paid to skills such as error prevention,[1] teamwork, leadership, situational awareness, decision-making, task management, and communication.[1,21-23] Although these skills are regularly taught in crew resource management courses in anesthesia, civil aviation, and oil exploration, they have not yet been taken seriously enough in surgery to be addressed explicitly in training. This is surprising, given the impact of nontechnical skills on patient safety.[22]

Another pitfall is that existing methods of assessing surgical trainees have been criticized as being subjective, inconsistent, or all too focused on quantity versus quality. Letters of recommendation provide highly subjective, and often incomplete, individual impressions of trainees' capabilities and can be easily influenced by the dynamics of personality. Personal logbooks record the number of procedures performed but provide little data on patient outcomes or technical skill. Logbooks document experience, not expertise. Even objective data such as professional examination scores assess factual knowledge but cannot evaluate how a trainee applies such knowledge to the day-to-day management of patients. Formal methods of assessing trainees' interactions with patients or ability to work in a team, such as Objective Structured Clinical Examinations or Non-Technical Skills for Surgeons, are infrequently used in the residency setting.[22]

So how can we determine if residents are receiving appropriate instruction on patient safety and developing practices conducive to minimizing errors? Central to any method of objective evaluation is a clear determination of the skills required for comprehensive surgical competence.

What is Important to Teach: Nontechnical Skill Development

Baldwin and colleagues offer a well-developed taxonomy of technical and nontechnical skills identified by 111 consultant surgeons in Europe considered valuable for a basic surgical trainee to develop. These priorities are divided into 5 distinct areas, listed in order of importance: technical skills such as proper handling of tissue and instruments; clinical skills with identifying acutely ill patients, carrying out thorough examinations, and documenting judiciously considered most important; teamwork; communication with patients and relatives; and application of knowledge.[21] McDonald and colleagues[24] interviewed 33 surgeons from a range of specialties including neurosurgery, orthopedic, and general and identified 7 characteristics of surgical excellence: commitment, self-belief, positive imagery, mental readiness, full focus, controlling distractions, and constructive evaluation. Another group showed correlation of better outcomes with high performance in behavioral markers such as mental readiness, cognitive flexibility, situational and safety awareness, anticipation, and team adaptation.[23] Of the 3 major readiness factors rated by surgeons—mental, technical, and physical—McDonald and colleagues[24] found that highly successful surgeons perform at an exceptional level largely because of the quality of their mental skills. Residents in surgery may benefit from systematic training in mental preparation.

Training Residents: a Focus on Patient Safety

Organizations such as the Accreditation Council for Graduate Medical Education (ACGME), the Institute of Healthcare Improvement (IHI), and the American College of Surgeons (ACS) have put significant emphasis on educating residents about patient safety.[1,25] The ACGME introduced the Clinical Learning Environment Review program, which provides the Sponsoring Institutions of residency programs with feedback on patient safety in hopes of improving how programs engage residents and fellows in learning to provide safe, high-quality patient care. The IHI has a well-recognized "Open School" online curriculum for residents to participate in and completion results in a Basic Certificate in Quality and Safety.[25] Finally, the ACS National Surgical Quality Improvement Program launched the Quality In-Training Initiative at its 2011 annual meeting. The program results from a collaboration between ACS and teaching hospitals to equip surgery residents with the skills needed to address quality in surgical patient care through data-driven initiatives. One initiative is the delivery of resident-specific 30-day outcome reports that can be used to facilitate the quality and safety dialogue between trainees and program directors.[26] Despite these organizational efforts as well as the recommendations of the Institute of Medicine, currently there is no nationally required resident curriculum specifically for patient safety, with teaching sites ultimately responsible for developing, implementing, and evaluating their own education programs.[27,28]

Most of the trainees have never been formally trained on patient preparation for surgical cases.[13] This suggests a gap in education that directly affects proper transition of care, and in turn, patient safety, but one that can easily be remedied. Options include didactic sessions on standardizing processes for preparation or simulation cases displaying the safety issues that can result from lack of preparation. Another approach is generally trying to allow residents an appropriate amount of notice by assigning cases, say, at the beginning of each week.

Although studies often look at mistakes leading to compromised patient safety, a singular focus on failure may not always be best for learning about the strategies needed to train residents to succeed; we must learn from successes as well.[23] As each residency program is unique in structure, this should involve broader dissemination of systems-based processes that work. For example, Putnam and colleagues have shown that combining an online safety curriculum (OC) with a series of physician-led, operative safety workshops (SW) may prove successful. Although the addition of an SW to the online component did not significantly improve overall perceptions of safety culture in all residents, senior residents participating in the SW demonstrated improved patient safety perceptions and had significantly better intraoperative safety behaviors than senior residents only participating in OC. This may suggest that future curricular enhancements could be training-level specific and require increased faculty involvement.[28]

Further, it follows principles of adult learning to involve residents in designing their own program-level or institution-wide patient safety programs. This includes processes around paging, sign-out, reporting and discussing errors, and procedural training and assessment. At Johns Hopkins, surgical chief residents developed 10 essential tools for effective sign-outs that are now used widely.[29] At University of Washington, a design team consisting of general surgery residents and faculty developed and validated an institution-wide computerized resident sign-out system with input of residents from 8 different services.[10] They were able to demonstrate improved quality and continuity of care and efficiency superior to telephone, video-based, or screen-based alternatives.[30]

As discussed, one key to enhancing trainees' roles in patient safety is standardization, and researchers continue to investigate methods to standardize content within the format of many day-to-day communication activities. Another key may lie in changing the overall training environment structure in and out of the operating room. Today, a significant portion of safety research focuses on perceptions of residents and staff about communication and teamwork in the operating room.[31] This body of work demonstrates that communication failures between residents and faculty are far more complex than simply the result of poor information exchange and more often relate to underlying hierarchical differences, anxiety about upward influence, role ambiguity, and interpersonal conflict.[32] Attending physicians are often unaware of house staff concerns about patient management issues, suggesting that residents need encouragement to open up and discuss their concerns with faculty.[33] Likewise, Coats and Burd[34] showed that fewer residents felt comfortable asking faculty to discuss their intraoperative decisions than was perceived by faculty members themselves. In an anonymous survey of surgery, orthopedic, and OBGYN residents and attending physicians, Belyansky and colleagues[31] found that although all attendings reported encouraging residents to question their intraoperative decision-making, only 55% of residents agreed. Furthermore, residents frequently did not agree with the attending's intraoperative management. Clearly a need exists for improved communication between the faculty and trainees.[34] This is of utmost importance, as collaboration between trainees and their superiors directly affect patient outcomes, and most of the residents and attendings can recall incidents where expression of concerns by residents had prevented an adverse outcome or where lack thereof resulted in complications.[35]

A Note on Simulation

Simulation-based surgical skills training (both technical and nontechnical) for students and residents can addresses several of the drawbacks associated with the traditional apprenticeship model to training.[36] Studies have shown simulator training can improve team and unit training, safety and quality initiatives,[37] decrease surgical times, improve basic surgical techniques, and optimize management of intraoperative and postoperative complications.[38,39] These educational initiatives should be of utmost importance during this era of increased vigilance for patient safety and quality improvement in health care.

Assessment of proficiency using standardized objective measurements is critical in improving the quality of surgical education. Several methods exist: questionnaires, Objective Structured Assessment of Technical Skills (OSATS), Global Rating Scale (GRS), Crowd-Sourced Assessment of Technical Skills (C-SATS), and direct objective metric tools. Questionnaires generate feedback from trainees regarding their personal evaluation of proficiency. Although practical and low-cost tools, questionnaires can have inherent shortcomings including subjectivity and difficulty in standardization. OSATS consist of a checklist of specific surgical maneuvers completed by observers to evaluate performance after the completion of simulation and to provide formative feedback during future simulations. GRS is another tool often used to complement OSATS to measure overall surgical skill as a comprehensive assessment including measures for nontechnical cognitive skills. C-SATS consists of a combination of OSATS and GRS completed by a decentralized, anonymous crowd of raters that may or may not have medical training.[36] Surprisingly, concordance between surgeon and crowd graders is high and may increase the accountability of outcomes by soliciting contributions from a larger community rather than strictly from medical professionals.[40]

SUMMARY

Mitigating risks of adverse events and ensuring a culture of safety throughout the health system involves strategies that span from revamping system-wide processes to training physicians and other care providers. There is generally significant inconsistency in perceptions of safety culture based on level of training, and it is imperative front-line workers such as learners are educated in patient safety principles and programs from the get-go. Medical students could benefit from the introduction of patient safety principles into their curricula, with existing modules or lessons in topics such as ethics. In addition, learning surgical patient safety principles should be emphasized on clinical rotations such as during time spent in the perioperative setting. Special focus should be placed on observing elements that influence team dynamics and success such as quality of leadership and communication both intraoperatively and during handoffs.

Despite recommendations from many national organizations, a standardized national curriculum in patient safety has not yet been developed for surgical residents. Furthermore, current methods for evaluating residents often overlook trainees' interactions with patients, leadership, and teamwork skills. Adopting these new focus areas into surgical training could entail wider adoption of components already in use by training programs combined with development of standardized simulation exercises and assessment instruments to more comprehensively evaluate both technical and nontechnical skills of surgical residents and further enhance safety of patients under their care, for both the present and the future.

CLINICS CARE POINTS

Pearls

- Emphasis on teamwork, operating room etiquette, effective communication, and following protocols during surgical clinical rotations should be a component of any patient safety curriculum for medical students.
- What entails thorough preparation for surgery and appropriate communication during transition of care should be emphasized early on in training so that medical students and young residents proceed with only the best habits.
- Simulation-based training-level–specific exercises can be used to target multiple facets of surgical patient safety education including development of nontechnical skills in addition to technical surgical skills.

Pitfalls

- Communication breakdown, a frequent contributor to adverse medical events, often occurs due to inconsistent handoff procedures.
- The lack of an objective, consistent safety curriculum and current hierarchical structure of residency programs leads to suppressed trainee voice and significant impact on patient outcomes.
- An online curriculum may not be adequate in training residents in surgical patient safety; workshops with increased faculty involvement and system-wide change toward standardized processes have a larger impact on patient safety culture.

DISCLOSURE

The authors have nothing to disclose.

REFERENCES

1. Putnam LR, Levy SM, Kellagher CM, et al. Surgical resident education in patient safety: where can we improve? J Surg Res 2015;199(2):308–13.
2. Greenberg CC, Regenbogen SE, Studdert DM, et al. Patterns of Communication Breakdowns Resulting in Injury to Surgical Patients. J Am Coll Surg 2007;204(4): 533–40.

3. World Health O. WHO patient safety curriculum guide for medical schools. Geneva (Switzerland): World Health Organization; 2009.

4. Leape LL, Brennan TA, Laird N, et al. The nature of adverse events in hospitalized patients. Results of the Harvard Medical Practice Study II. N Engl J Med 1991; 324(6):377–84.

5. Kohn LT, Corrigan J, Donaldson MS. To err is human: building a safer health system, vol. 6. Washington, DC: National academy press; 2000.

6. Commission J. Patient safety systems (PS). Comprehensive Accreditation Manual for Hospitals. 2017. Available at: https://www.jointcommission.org/patient_safety_systems_chapter_for_the_hospital_program/. 3. Accessed May 4, 2020.

7. Pimentel MPT, Choi S, Fiumara K, et al. Safety culture in the operating room: variability among perioperative healthcare workers. J Patient Saf 2017. https://doi.org/10.1097/PTS.0000000000000385.

8. Christian CK, Gustafson ML, Roth EM, et al. A prospective study of patient safety in the operating room. Surgery 2006;139(2):159–73.

9. Lingard L, Espin S, Whyte S, et al. Communication failures in the operating room: an observational classification of recurrent types and effects. Qual Saf Health Care 2004;13(5):330–4.

10. Van Eaton EG, Horvath KD, Lober WB, et al. Organizing the transfer of patient care information: the development of a computerized resident sign-out system. Surgery 2004;136(1):5–13.

11. Petersen LA, Brennan TA, O'Neil AC, et al. Does housestaff discontinuity of care increase the risk for preventable adverse events? Ann Intern Med 1994;121(11): 866–72.

12. Davenport DL, Henderson WG, Mosca CL, et al. Risk-adjusted morbidity in teaching hospitals correlates with reported levels of communication and collaboration on surgical teams but not with scale measures of teamwork climate, safety climate, or working conditions. J Am Coll Surg 2007;205(6):778–84.

13. Mundschenk M-B, Odom EB, Ghosh TD, et al. Are residents prepared for surgical cases? implications in patient safety and education. J Surg Educ 2018;75(2): 403–8.

14. Walton M, Woodward H, Van Staalduinen S, et al. Republished paper: The WHO patient safety curriculum guide for medical schools. Postgrad Med J 2011; 87(1026):317–21.

15. Walton MM, Shaw T, Barnet S, et al. Developing a national patient safety education framework for Australia. Qual Saf Health Care 2006;15(6):437–42.

16. WHO Multi-professional Patient Safety Curriculum Guide. 2019. Available at: https://www.who.int/patientsafety/education/mp_curriculum_guide/en/. Accessed May 4, 2020.

17. Leape LL. Error in medicine. JAMA 1994;272(23):1851–7.

18. Goldie J. Review of ethics curricula in undergraduate medical education. Med Educ 2000;34(2):108–19.

19. Goldie JGS. The detrimental ethical shift towards cynicism: can medical educators help prevent it? Med Educ 2004;38(3):232–4.

20. Wohlauer MV, George B, Lawrence PF, et al. Review of Influential Articles in Surgical Education: 2002–2012. J Grad Med Educ 2013;5(2):219–26.

21. Baldwin PJ, Paisley AM, Paterson Brown S. Consultant surgeons' opinion of the skills required of basic surgical trainees. Br J Surg 1999;86(8):1078–82.

22. Yule S, Flin R, Paterson-Brown S, et al. Non-technical skills for surgeons in the operating room: A review of the literature. Surgery 2006;139(2):140–9.

23. Carthey J, de Leval MR, Wright DJ, et al. Behavioural markers of surgical excellence. Saf Sci 2003;41(5):409–25.
24. McDonald J, Orlick T, Letts M. Mental readiness in surgeons and its links to performance excellence in surgery. J Pediatr Orthop 1995;15(5):691–7.
25. Overview: IHI - Institute for Healthcare Improvement. 2020. Available at: http://www.ihi.org/education/ihiopenschool/overview/Pages/default.aspx. Accessed 2020.
26. Sakran JV, Hoffman RL, Ko C, et al. The ACS NSQIp quality in-training initiative: educating residents to ensure the future of optimal surgical care. Bull Am Coll Surg 2013;98(11):30–5.
27. Accreditation Council for Graduate Medical Education: Clinical Learning Environment Review Program. Available at: https://www.acgme.org/What-We-Do/Initiatives/Clinical-Learning-Environment-Review-CLER. Accessed February 21, 2020.
28. Putnam LR, Pham DH, Ostovar-Kermani TG, et al. How should surgical residents be educated about patient safety: a pilot randomized controlled trial. J Surg Educ 2016;73(4):660–7.
29. Kemp CD, Bath JM, Berger J, et al. The top 10 list for a safe and effective sign-out. Arch Surg 2008;143(10):1008–10.
30. Van Eaton EG, Horvath KD, Lober WB, et al. A randomized, controlled trial evaluating the impact of a computerized rounding and sign-out system on continuity of care and resident work hours. J Am Coll Surg 2005;200(4):538–45.
31. Belyansky I, Martin TR, Prabhu AS, et al. Poor resident-attending intraoperative communication may compromise patient safety. J Surg Res 2011;171(2):386–94.
32. Sutcliffe KM, Lewton E, Rosenthal MM. Communication failures: an insidious contributor to medical mishaps. Acad Med 2004;79(2):186–94.
33. Shreves JG, Moss AH. Residents' ethical disagreements with attending physicians: an unrecognized problem. Acad Med 1996;71(10):1103–5.
34. Coats RD, Burd RS. Intraoperative communication of residents with faculty: perception versus reality. J Surg Res 2002;104(1):40–5.
35. Barzallo Salazar MJ, Minkoff H, Bayya J, et al. Influence of surgeon behavior on trainee willingness to speak up: a randomized controlled trial. J Am Coll Surg 2014;219(5):1001–7.
36. Atesok K, Satava RM, Marsh JL, et al. Measuring surgical skills in simulation-based training. J Am Acad Orthop Surg 2017;25(10):665–72.
37. Satin AJ. Simulation in Obstetrics. Obstet Gynecol 2018;132(1):199–209.
38. Waterman BR, Martin KD, Cameron KL, et al. Simulation training improves surgical proficiency and safety during diagnostic shoulder arthroscopy performed by residents. Orthopedics 2016;39(3):e479–85.
39. Tannyhill RJ 3rd, Jensen OT. Computer simulation and maxillary all-on-four surgery. Oral Maxillofac Surg Clin North Am 2019;31(3):497–504.
40. Holst D, Kowalewski TM, White LW, et al. Crowd-sourced assessment of technical skills: differentiating animate surgical skill through the wisdom of crowds. J Endourol 2015;29(10):1183–8.

Moving?

Make sure your subscription moves with you!

To notify us of your new address, find your **Clinics Account Number** (located on your mailing label above your name), and contact customer service at:

Email: journalscustomerservice-usa@elsevier.com

800-654-2452 (subscribers in the U.S. & Canada)
314-447-8871 (subscribers outside of the U.S. & Canada)

Fax number: 314-447-8029

Elsevier Health Sciences Division
Subscription Customer Service
3251 Riverport Lane
Maryland Heights, MO 63043